Clinical Aspects of Albumin

Clinical Aspects of Albumin

edited by

S.H. Yap

St. Radboud Hospital, University of Nijmegen and Albert Einstein College of Medicine, New York

C.L.H. Majoor

St. Radboud Hospital, University of Nijmegen

J.H.M. van Tongeren

St. Radboud Hospital, University of Nijmegen

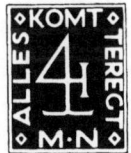

1978

Martinus Nijhoff Medical Division

The Hague/Boston/London

ISBN-13: 978-94-009-9746-2   *e-ISBN-13: 978-94-009-9744-8*

DOI: 10.1007/978-94-009-9744-8

Photoset in Malta

Table of contents

List of contributors

E.J. Ariëns, M.D., Ph.D., Professor of Pharmacology, Pharmacological Institute, University of Nijmegen, Geert Grooteplein Noord 21, Nijmegen, The Netherlands

J.C.L.H. Benneker, Pharmacist, Department of Clinical Pharmacy, St. Radboud Hospital, Nijmegen, The Netherlands

H. Bloemendal, Ph.D., Professor of Biochemistry, Department of Biochemistry, University of Nijmegen, Geert Grooteplein Noord 21, Nijmegen, The Netherlands

O.J.J. Cluysenaer, M.D., Department of Medicine, Division of Gastroenterology, St. Radboud Hospital, University of Nijmegen, Nijmegen, The Netherlands. Present address: St. Elisabeth Hospital, Amersfoort, The Netherlands

H.G. van Eijk, Ph.D., Department of Chemical Pathology, Dijkzigt Hospital, Erasmus University, Rotterdam, The Netherlands

J. Gerbrandy, M.D., Professor of Medicine, Department of Medicine I, Dijkzigt Hospital, Erasmus University, Rotterdam, The Netherlands

R.J.A. Goris, M.D., Department of General Surgery, St. Radboud Hospital, University of Nijmegen, Nijmegen, The Netherlands

Y.A. Hekster, Pharmacist, Department of Clinical Pharmacy, St. Radboud Hospital, Nijmegen, The Netherlands

S. Jarnum, M.D., Medical Department P, Division of Gastroenterology, Rigshospitalet, Copenhagen, Denmark

K.B. Jensen, M.D., Medical Department P, Division of Gastroenterology, Rigshospitalet, Copenhagen, Denmark

E. van der Kleijn, Ph.D., Director of Department of Clinical Pharmacy, St. Radboud Hospital, Nijmegen, The Netherlands

H.W. Krijnen, Ph.D., Central Laboratory of the Netherlands Red Cross Blood Transfusion Service, Amsterdam, The Netherlands

C.B.H. Lamers, M.D., Department of Medicine, Division of Gastroenterology, St. Radboud Hospital, University of Nijmegen, The Netherlands

R.W.M.M. Langenhoff, Department of Clinical Pharmacy, St. Radboud Hospital, Nijmegen, The Netherlands

C.L.H. Majoor, M.D., Professor of Medicine, Department of Medicine, St. Radboud Hospital, University of Nijmegen, Nijmegen, The Netherlands

P.H.M. de Mulder, M.D., Department of Medicine, St. Radboud Hospital, University of Nijmegen, Nijmegen, The Netherlands

M. Oratz, Ph.D., Assistant Chief Department of Nuclear Medicine, Veterans Administration Hospital, Adjunct Professor of Biochemistry, New York University Dental Center, New York, NY 10010, U.S.A.

M.A. Rothschild, M.D., Chief Department of Nuclear Medicine, Veterans Administration Hospital, Professor of Medicine, New York University School of Medicine, New York, NY 10010, U.S.A.

S.S. Schreiber, M.D., Attending Physician Veterans Administration Hospital, Professor of Medicine, New York University School of Medicine, New York, NY 10010, U.S.A.

D.A. Shafritz, M.D., Associate Professor of Medicine and Cell Biology, Albert Einstein College of Medicine of Yeshiva University, 1300 Morris Park Avenue, Bronx, NY 10461, U.S.A.

A.M. Simonis, Pharmacological Institute, University of Nijmegen, Greet Grooteplein Noord 21, Nijmegen, The Netherlands

S.J. Smith, M.D., Department of Medicine I, Dijkzigt Hospital, Erasmus University, Rotterdam, The Netherlands. Present address: Diakonessenhuis, Paramaribo, Suriname

A.M. Stadhouders, Ph.D., Director Division of Electron Microscopy, University of Nijmegen Medical School, Geert Grooteplein Zuid 24, Nijmegen, The Netherlands

R.K. Strair, Ph.D., Albert Einstein College of Medicine of Yeshiva University, 1300 Morris Park Avenue, Bronx, NY 10461, U.S.A.

J.H.M. van Tongeren, M.D., Department of Medicine, Division of Gastroenterology, St. Radboud Hospital, University of Nijmegen, Nijmegen, The Netherlands

S.H. Yap, M.D., Department of Medicine, Division of Gastroenterology, St. Radboud Hospital, University of Nijmegen, Nijmegen, and Albert Einstein College of Medicine of Yeshiva University, 1300 Morris Park Avenue, Bronx. NY 10461, U.S.A.

J.B. Zuidgeest, Department of Clinical Pharmacy, St. Radboud Hospital, Nijmegen, The Netherlands

Preface

Albumin is the most abundant serum protein produced by the liver. In clinical practice the serum level of albumin continues to be used as an important marker of the presence, progress or of the improvement of many diseases, even though it is the complex end result of synthesis, degradation and distribution between intra- and extravascular space.

The clinical history of albumin began as early as in 1837, when Ancell first recognized "albumen" and noted that this protein is needed for transport functions, for maintaining fluidity of the vascular system and for the prevention of edema. However, the important physiological properties of serum proteins and their role in the regulation of the oncotic pressure were demonstrated later by the physiologist E.H. Starling in 1895. In 1917 the clinician A.A. Epstein first described the edema in patients with the nephrotic syndrome as being a result of a very low level of serum albumin. Although the determination of serum albumin concentration became more popular after Howe in 1921 introduced the technique of separation of serum globulins from albumin by sodium sulfate, the first preparations of human serum albumin were made available for clinical use in only 1941 by the development of plasma fractionation by Cohn and his coworkers at Harvard Medical School. By using albumin labelled with radioactive iodine for clinical research, as introduced by Sterling in 1951, and by the development of the ^{14}C-carbonate method by McFarlane and Reeve in 1963 to measure albumin synthesis rate directly in vivo, it has become possible to study the regulation of albumin metabolism.

The purpose of this book is to present current concepts concerning biochemical, physiological, and pathophysiological factors regulating the synthesis, distribution and degradation of albumin, and the disorders that may produce abnormalities in albumin synthesis, catabolism and external loss. Since concentrated human serum albumin is used frequently in clinical practice, its applications in hypoproteinemia and in the treatment of shock are discussed in the second part of the book. In this regard the role of albumin in the maintenance of colloid osmotic pressure and in the transport function is also presented. This book gives in more detail the texts of papers presented at a Symposium on Metabolism, Function and Clinical Use of Albumin, held at the Medical Faculty, University of Nijmegen, October 1977.

The editors hope that this publication will be of interest to all concerned with problems of albumin metabolism in clinical medicine. We are much obliged to the authors of all papers in this Symposium for their important contributions. We wish also to thank the Board of the Medical Faculty, University of Nijmegen, Institut Mérieux, and The Central Laboratory of The Netherlands Red Cross Blood Transfusion Service, Amsterdam, for their financial supports in organizing this Symposium.

S.H. YAP
C.L.H. MAJOOR
J.H.M. VAN TONGEREN
Department of Medicine
St. Radboud Hospital
University of Nijmegen

1. The mechanism of protein biosynthesis

H. BLOEMENDAL

The complicated pathways on which protein biosynthesis is based can be summarized in a simple schematic representation.

$$\text{DNA} \xrightarrow{\text{transcription}} \text{RNA} \xrightarrow{\text{translation}} \text{protein}$$

This means that messenger RNA (mRNA) molecules transfer genetic information from DNA to electron-dense cell particles, the ribosomes for the synthesis of polypeptide chains. The linear sequence of amino acids in a polypeptide chain corresponds to a linear sequence of nucleotides (in mRNA) consisting of three nucleotides each (the so-called codons) that determine which of the 20 different amino acids will be inserted into the polypeptide chain to be synthesized. A complementary sequence of the codon is found in another class of RNAs that are involved in the *transfer* of the activated amino acids to the ribosome and therefore are called tRNA.

The second scheme represents the major steps involved in the biosynthetic process *per se*.

I) Initiation
II) Elongation
III) Termination

In order to get the correct protein the reading of mRNA has to be started in such a way that the correct phase of the message is maintained. This is shown for a fragment of mRNA consisting of 12 nucleotides.

correct reading: Met Phe Ser Val
                    ___ ___ ___ ___
                    A UG UUU UCU GUA
                       ___ ___ ___
out of phase: Val Phe Cys

In this example not only the colinearity of messenger and polypeptide but also the so-called degeneracy of the genetic code is visualized. Degeneracy means that most amino acids can be represented by more than one codon (compare in our example valine which is encoded by GUA and GUU). Having the foregoing in mind, one can easily conclude that the message has to begin on a fixed point on the mRNA that corresponds to the first amino acid of the protein.

INITIATION

It was known for a rather long time that the synthesis of a protein starts at the NH$_2$ terminus. However, two discoveries in particular contributed to the ultimate understanding of correct initiation. First the observation that all proteins are synthesized beginning with formyl-methionine, at least in prokaryotes. In some stage of the biosynthetic process the formyl group is released and in most cases also the terminal methionyl residue is removed. Only incidentally methionine remains at the N-terminus of the protein. In our studies on lens proteins we found that α-crystallin is such an exception (1). The reason why in rare cases methionine resists cleavage is unclear.

The second important finding relative to the initiation was the discovery of a transfer RNA species (tRNA$_f^{Met}$) specific for a methionine molecule which could be formylated. In this respect α-crystallin is very illustrative. In each of the polypeptide chains of this protein only two methionine residues occur; one in N-terminal position, the other one internally (compare Fig. 1). We could easily demonstrate in a cell-free system derived from isolated calf lenses that two different tRNA species were required for the correct insertion of the methionine residues. Here it has to be kept in mind that the N-terminal methionine in eukaryotes can be formylated in vitro but does not exist as such *in situ*.

The actual initiation point of protein biosynthesis is governed by a number of protein factors. Although it was believed for some time that three of those proteins are required, thorough studies by Schreier and Staehelin (2) and by the group of Anderson (3) revealed the existence of at least 7 different initiation factors in eukaryotes. The rather complex initiation reaction is represented in a simplified way for a bacterial protein (Fig. 2).

The peptide chain can be started after binding of the small ribosomal subunit to a specific region of the mRNA where an AUG codon is situated. This binding requires the so-called initiation factor F$_3$. The complex can

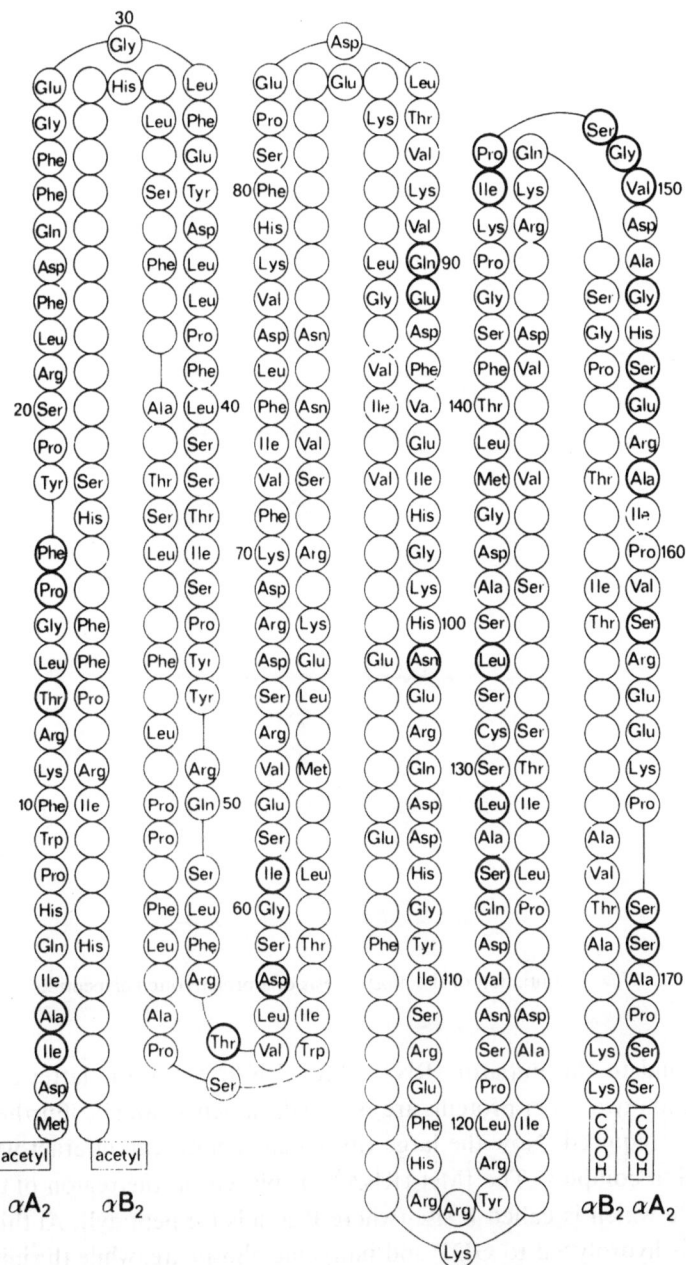

Fig. 1. Primary structure of the lens protein α-crystallin. Note the 2 methionine residues in the polypeptide chains (position 1 and 138, A chain; position 1 and 64, B chain, respectively). Blank circles in the B chain represent identical amino acid residues as compared to the A chain.

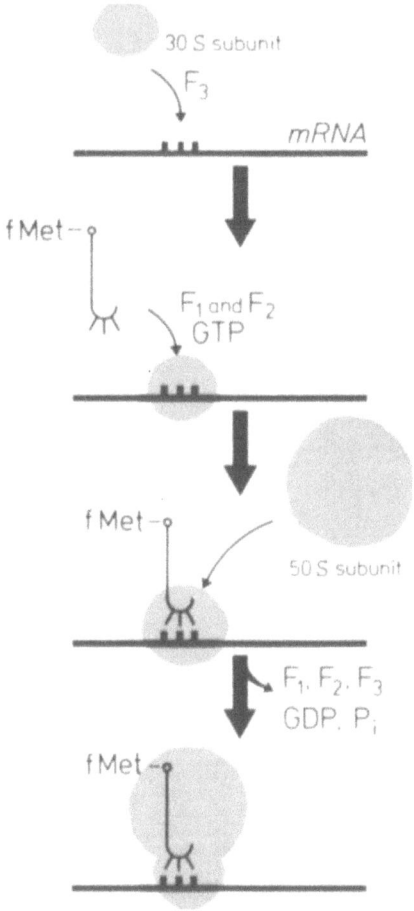

Fig. 2. Initiation of the biosynthesis of a prokaryotic polypeptide.

then bind to the initiator tRNA: fMet-tRNA$_f^{Met}$. For the latter complex formation two other proteins are essential, namely F_1 and F_2. Furthermore GTP is required. Now the large ribosomal subunit can interact with the initiation complex. The fMet-tRNA$_f^{Met}$ is placed on the region of the 50S particle which is called P site (where P stands for peptidyl). At this stage GTP is hydrolyzed to GDP and inorganic phosphate, while the initiation factors are released. The various stages summarized above lead to a 70S ribosome bound to messenger RNA with the initiation codon A UG in the proper position.

ELONGATION

The amino acids are polymerized on the ribosome by peptide bond formation. Since for the formation of each peptide bond two amino acids are required, a minimum of two sites for amino acids should be present on the ribosome. Experimental evidence supports the concept that each ribosome can accommodate the binding of two tRNA molecules. The P site which is also designated as donor site has been mentioned before. It binds the tRNA molecule to which the N-terminal end of the growing peptide chain is attached (see Fig. 3). The other site, called amino-acyl, acceptor or A site, binds a tRNA molecule which carries the amino acid to be inserted next. Thus peptide bond formation occurs by interaction between the free terminal COOH-group of the growing peptide chain and the free α-NH$_2$ group of the amino acid attached to the tRNA at the A site. Before the following amino acid can be inserted, the tRNA carrying

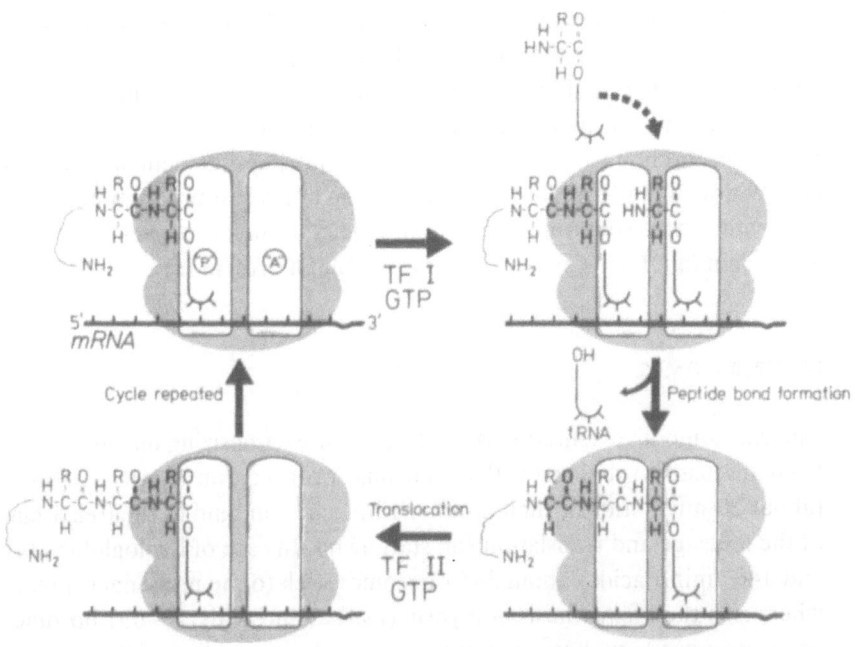

Fig. 3. Elongation of a polypeptide during the process of biosynthesis.

the polypeptide chain has to be transferred from the A site to the P site. This movement is called translocation.

Also for the process of elongation specific protein factors are required. A protein called transfer factor I (TF I) interacts with the amino acid carrying tRNA and GTP to place the tRNA in the correct position on the ribosome. GTP is hydrolyzed to GDP and inorganic phosphate in this reaction. The formation of the peptide bond is catalyzed by a protein called peptidyl transferase, which has been proven to be one of the numerous proteins of the large ribosomal subunit.

Another protein, transfer factor II (TF II), is involved in the translocation reaction. Also this process is accompanied by hydrolysis of a GTP molecule to GDP and inorganic phosphate.

TERMINATION

In the genetic code three of the 64 existing codons do not correspond to any known amino acid. It could be shown that these codons UAA, UAG and UGA are the signals for chain termination. Termination involves the release of the last transfer RNA molecule from the ribosome. Evidence has been provided that also in this last step of protein biosynthesis specific protein factors are involved that recognize the termination codons and hydrolyze the bond between the complete polypeptide chain and the last tRNA molecule (4). Failure to terminate may lead to production of protein with extra, sometimes structurally deleterious amino acids. For example hemoglobin "Constant Spring" is such a protein (5).

POLYRIBOSOMES

The ribosome as essential part of the protein-synthesizing machinery has been discussed previously. If a ribosome proceeds on a mRNA strand (about 30 nucleotides), then another ribosome can bind to the free 5′ end of the message and translation can start again. In case of hemoglobin (141 and 146 amino acids) about 3–5 ribosomes stick to the messenger thread, whereas in the biosynthesis of myosin (2000 amino acids) 50–60 ribosomes per messenger have been observed. Although the reading of the message cannot be repeated infinitely, a rather long life-span has been observed for some messengers in eukaryotic cells like reticulocytes and lens cells. The clusters of ribosomes called polyribosomes can be visualized in the electron microscope (Fig. 4). In most eukaryotic cells the polyribosomes occur in two classes, i.e. either attached to membrane structures (endoplasmic reticulum) or lying free in the cytoplasm. Membrane-bound ribosomes are thought to be the sites of synthesis of proteins necessary for export from the cell (6).

POST-TRANSLATIONAL MODIFICATIONS

Protein biosynthesis is not only the translation of the genetic message. Several modifications of the primary translation product occurring either shortly after initiation or upon its release from the ribosome may represent additional important steps in the formation of the protein. Phosphorylation of serine residues (7), hydroxylation of proline in collagen (8) or the addi-

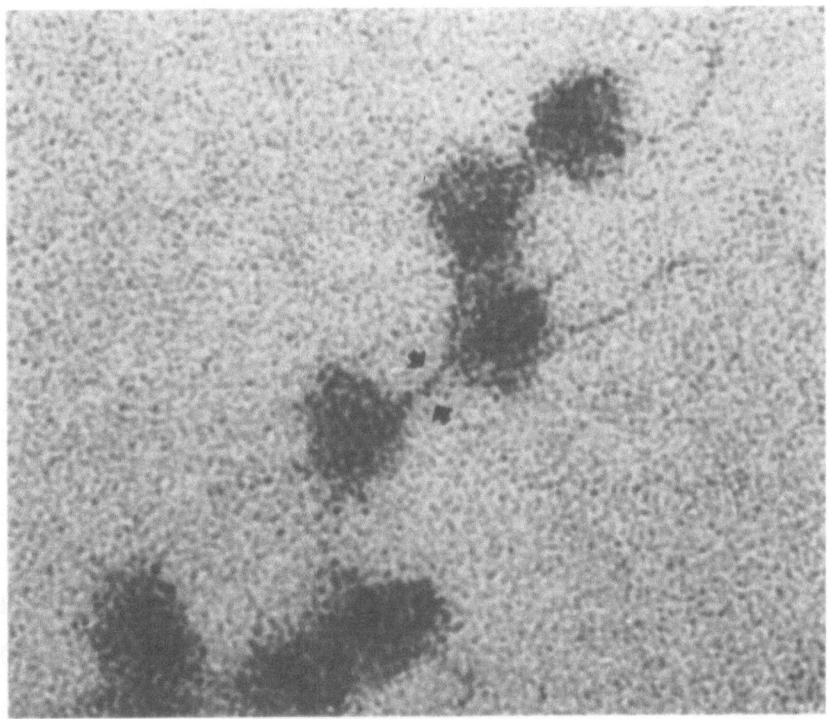

Fig. 4. Electron micrograph of polyribosomes isolated from calf lens tissue. The arrows point to the messenger. Magnification 480,000 ×.

tion of lipids (9) or carbohydrates (10) are well-known post-translational changes of the newly synthesized polypeptide. Another frequently occurring modification is the N-terminal acetylation of eukaryotic and viral proteins (Fig. 1). We studied this phenomenon with α-crystallin and found that acetylation takes place while the polypeptide chain is still on the ribosome (1). The meaning of the modifications mentioned is far from being understood. In case of acetylation it may provide an efficient protection against enzymatic degradation starting from the NH_2 terminal end.

Whereas in earlier biochemical work tissue slices were used to carry out, at least for a period, protein biosynthesis in vitro, more recently cell-free incubation systems have been prepared from various tissues which respond to the addition of exogenous messengers (11). For instance isolated albumin messenger RNA can direct the synthesis of albumin in lysates from reticulocytes, wheat germ or ascites tumor cells. An alternative is the injection of purified messenger preparations into living oocytes from Xenopus laevis (12).

In many cases the newly formed protein is indistinguishable from the native product, although the cell-free systems may lack the ability to process precursor polypeptides to the final proteins.

REFERENCES

1. Bloemendal H: The vertebrate eye lens. Science 197:127–138, 1977.
2. Schreier MH, Staehelin T: 24th Mosbach Coll, Springer Verlag, Heidelberg, 1973, p 335.
3. Anderson WF, Bosch L, Cohn WE, et al: International symposium on protein synthesis. FEBS Lett 76: 1–10, 1977.
4. Capecchi MR: Polypeptide chain termination in vitro: Isolation of a release factor. Proc Natl Acad Sci USA 58:1144–1151, 1967.
5. Chegg JB, Weatherhall DJ and Milner PF: Haemoglobin Constant Sprint – a chain termination mutant. Nature 234:337–340, 1971.
6. Bloemendal H, Benedetti EL, Bont WS: Preparation and characterization of free- and membrane-bound polysomes. In: Methods in Enzymology vol XXX, New York-London, Academic Press, 1974, pp 313–325.
7. Jergil B: Protein kinase from rainbow-trout-testis ribosomes. Eur J Biochem 28: 546–554, 1972.
8. Udenfriend S: Formation of hydroxyproline in collagen. Science 152:1335–1340, 1966.
9. Scanu AM, Wisdom C: Serum lipoproteins structure and function. Ann Rev Biochem 41:703–730, 1972.
10. Winterburn PJ, Phelps CF: The significance of glycosylated proteins. Nature (Lond) 236:147–151, 1972.
11. Berns AJM, Bloemendal H: Cytoplasmic messenger RNA. In: Handbook of Genetics, vol 5, Molecular Genetics, New York, Plenum Press, 1976, pp 267–305.
12. Gurdon JB, Lane CD, Woodland HR, et al: Use of frog eggs and oocytes for the study of messenger RNA and its translation in living cells. Nature 233:177–182, 1971.

2. Intracellular transport and secretion of proteins

A.M. STADHOUDERS

INTRODUCTION

Ultrastructural studies have revealed a complex intracellular differentiation of eukaryotic cells. The interior is subdivided into a number of subcellular compartments, bounded by lipoprotein membranes with the inability of macromolecules to freely cross these membrane barriers. The multitude of processes which together account for the functioning of the living cell occur within these compartments and both on and in the limiting membranes. The integration of the processes occurring in different compartments into a coherent whole is facilitated by the presence in the barriers delineating the compartments, of special mechanisms for controlling the selective entry of substrates, the exit of products, and the transmembrane movements of regulatory substances and cofactors.

The high degree of subcellular compartmentation is of considerable benefit for the cell. The biosynthesis of many cellular constituents and their degradation occur in different compartments. The concentration of metabolites and enzymes of particular pathways in a small fraction of the total space allows efficient interaction whereas these pathways can at the same time and to a large extent remain isolated from competing or opposing reactions.

In view of the basic organization of eukaryotic cells, the story of secretion is largely the story of how the several compartments involved in the secretory process communicate with each other and/or with the extracellular environment.

GENERAL ASPECTS OF SECRETION

Secretion has been recognized in recent years as an important activity in a wide variety of cells. Many secretions, like plasma proteins, lipoproteins, digestive enzyms, etc., are macromolecular. Other cells, however, secrete small and charged molecules, such as catecholamines, histamine and acetylcholine. It is not likely to expect that either of these two types of molecules can freely pass the plasma membrane. Their release from the appropriate secretory cell as a rule occurs only in response to specific stimuli. Moreover, this release is usually not accompanied by an appreciable liberation of cytoplasmic matrix substances (such as glycolytic enzymes).

In order to explain these facts one must either assume special molecular mechanisms for transporting each individual secretory product through the plasma membrane or the ability to segregate molecules destined for export from material for domestic use with the possibility to release the segregated molecules when necessary or desired.

Arguments in favour of the latter mechanism have now emerged from studies of a wide variety of tissues. This mechanism or some slight variant of it, appears relevant for the process of synthesis, intracellular transport, storage and extrusion out of the cell of a wide range of secretory materials of diverse biological functions.

BASIC SECRETORY PATHWAY

The sequence of steps in intracellular protein transport and secretion has been studied most extensively in the pancreatic exocrine cell. Much of our current understanding of the nature of secretion as a cellular activity is derived from studies of this cell type.

Cells which are specialized for secretion show several structural features in common. The pancreatic exocrine cells in particular are markedly polarized, both from the functional and the structural point of view. The manufacture of secretory proteins occurs at the base of the cell and the secretion of these products into the acinar lumen occurs at the cell top.

Fig. 1 illustrates the basic secretory pathway for export proteins in such cells: bound polyribosomes – rough endoplasmic reticulum – smooth surfaced vesicles – Golgi cisternae – condensing vacuoles – storage vesicles – luminal membrane.

An outstanding aspect of this intracellular transport route is that, after their synthesis, the exportable proteins are at all times kept within membrane-bound channels or vesicles, i.e. the export proteins follow a membrane-bound intracellular route.

Palade (1) has distinguished six successive steps or operations in the

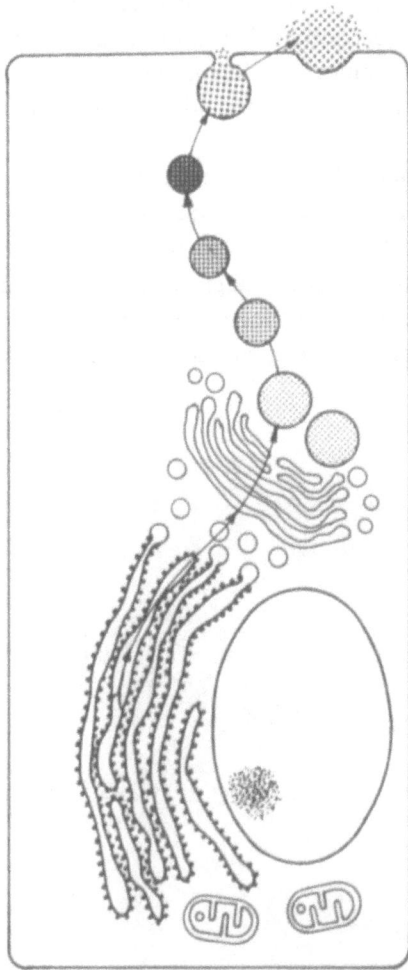

Fig. 1. Diagram of the basic secretory pathway. Export proteins are segregated into the rough ER cisternae, transported into the Golgi complex, concentrated in storage granules and released by exocytosis.

secretory cycle: (I) synthesis, (II) segregation, (III) transport, (VI) concentration, (V) storage and (VI) discharge. We will follow this scheme further below.

SYNTHESIS

For a description of the mechanism of protein synthesis, the reader is referred to the contribution of Dr. Bloemendal (Chapter I). Only some aspect of "compartmentation" of the protein-synthesizing machinery will be considered here. It has long been recognized that in most eukaryotic cells there are two populations of ribosomes, one free in the cell sap and another associated with the membranes of the endoplasmic reticulum (ER).

Moreover, it is a common finding that cells secreting proteins have abundant ER membranes studded with ribosomes. For example, in the exocrine pancreas cell, the rough ER accounts for 30–50% of the total cell volume (Fig. 2). The liver cell also has a well developed rough-surfaced ER and half the protein it synthesizes is exported in the form of plasma proteins. Cells, which retain their synthesized proteins (e.g. reticulocytes), show few

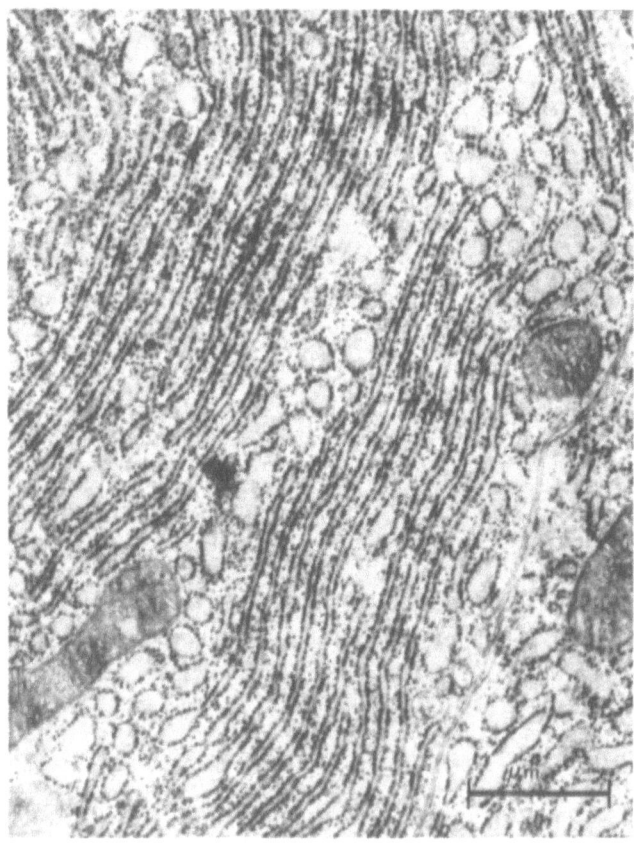

Fig. 2. Closely packed ER cisternae with bound ribosomes in an exocrine pancreatic cell.

membrane-bound ribosomes but have many ribosomes lying free in the cytoplasm.

These findings have led to the concept that proteins for export are made on membrane-bound ribosomes, whereas retained proteins are made on free ribosomes.

There is a considerable biochemical support now for this concept mainly derived from studies which analyzed the directional discharge of polypeptides synthesized in vivo and in vitro on rough ER. It seems justified to generalize the conclusion that proteins destined for export are synthesized on bound ribosomes.

However, the reverse (proteins synthesized on bound polysomes are all exported from the cell) is not true. The liver cell is interesting in this point since experiments have shown that proteins, synthesized by bound polysomes, can also internally be transported to the inner compartment of other organelles. An example is the enzym-protein catalase which is a component of the liver peroxisomes. The same may apply to the various hydrolytic enzymes which populate the lysosomes. To some extent, therefore, these organelles may be thought of as "stay-at-home" secretory granules. Proteins falling into this latter category also include those membrane proteins which form the tightly bound class of integral proteins or which are deposited asymmetrically towards the noncytoplasmic face of ER membranes.

Whether transfer of nascent polypeptides across membranes is the underlying feature common to *all* proteins synthesized on bound ribosomes remains still to be determined. It has been suggested, for example, that a large fraction of the proteins synthesized by rough ER in non-secretory tissues is released from bound ribosomes directly to the cytosol (2). Regarding the subject of this symposium, some evidence has been presented, based on cytochemical observations in rat liver, that newly formed albumin molecules may be released from bound ribosomes directly into the cytosol (3).

SEGREGATION

The synthesis of the secretory polypeptide chains by bound polysomes is "vectorial" and results in the segregation of the newly synthesized proteins in the cisternal space of the rough ER.

This has been demonstrated for example for the synthesis of serum albumin in the liver and for amylase synthesis in the pancreatic cells by exploiting the impermeability of "microsomal" vesicles and the ability of puromycin to prematurely induce release of growing polypeptide chains from ribosomes. Microsomal vesicles, which arise from the ER upon homogenization of the tissue, are produced with their ribosome-loaded cytoplasmic surface to the exterior. Their interior is the in vitro equivalent of the ER cisternal space. Such vesicles, when isolated from a secretory tissue which has been exposed to a very short pulse of labelled amino acids, carry radioactive polypeptide chains on their ribosomes. These chains represent proteins whose translation was not completed at the time of homogenization. When the microsomes are treated with puromycin, most of the released chains are trapped within the vesicles and are liberated only when the membranes are disrupted. It appears that the proteins to be secreted do cross the ER-membranes early in their migration. The nature of the mechanism which is responsible for directing the polypeptide chains in the cisternal cavity is uncertain. It is known that ribosomes interact with the ER-membranes via their large subunits and also that the discharge across the membrane occurs through a site of passage which is close to or at the ribosome membrane junction. It has therefore been proposed that the nascent polypeptide grows within the large ribosomal subunit in a space which can become continuous with the cisternal space through a passageway in the membrane, which is either a temporary or a permanent feature of the membrane (Fig. 3a). In this view segregation is the result of vectorial transport of the newly synthesized polypeptide from the large ribosomal subunit. That the nascent polypeptides become directly associated with the underlying ER membranes was demonstrated in a study on the effects of proteolytic enzymes on the nascent polypeptides of rough microsomes, labeled in vitro (4). Mild proteolysis caused extensive removal of ribosomes but did not lead to complete digestion of the nascent chains. Instead, sufficiently long polypeptides were cleaved into two main classes of fragments, both of which were largely protected from proteolysis. The carboxyl-terminal ends of nascent polypeptides were removed with the detached ribosomes; the amino-terminal portions were retained in the denuded microsomes.

It would be of considerable interest to learn how the extra-ribosomal segment of the nascent polypeptide chain interacts with the microsomal membrane. Recent findings indicate that sufficiently long nascent chains tightly anchor the ribosomes to the membrane (5). This suggests a more intimate relationship between polypeptide chain and membrane than would be expected from a simple hole under the ribosome.

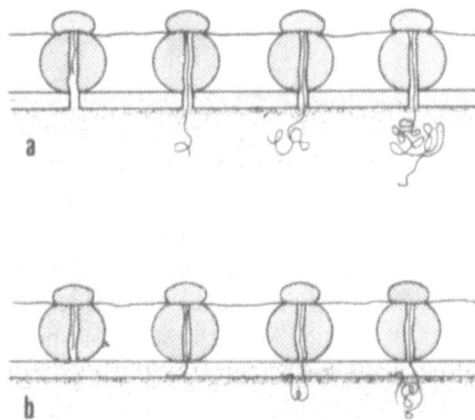

Fig. 3. Diagram of the vectorial discharge of nascent polypeptides across rough ER membranes, emphasizing (3a) passage through a hole in the large ribosomal subunit and the underlying ER membrane, (3b) the insertion of the amino-terminal end of the polypeptide chain into the membrane and subsequent folding of the chain as the driving force for transfer across the membrane.

In the "signal peptide" hypothesis of Blobel and Sabatini (6) a peptide portion, coded for by the 5′-phosphate end of the messenger RNA-chain through a still-to-be discovered recognition feature, directs this signal peptide into the vesicular membrane, followed by the growing chain. It may be hypothesized that the initial interaction of the nascent polypeptides with the membrane (Fig. 3b) results from the hydrophobic bounding between a nonpolar amino-terminal end of the chain and the membrane, or from other interactions determined by pertinent binding information contained in the amino-terminal sequences of the nascent chain. In this connection, it is important to emphasize that the vectorial discharge is passive in that it is non-enzymic and independent of the presence of ATP.

The emprisonment of the polypeptide chain in the ER cisternae most likely is the consequence of alterations of the peptide chains through enzymatic systems of the ER-membranes. The polypeptides are modified by processes such as hydroxylation, glycosidation, disulfide bridge formation, addition of carbohydrate or lipide residues and formation of disulfide cross-links. All these modifying operations are expected to affect directly or indirectly the tertiary structure, thus rendering the protein impermeant and their segregation irreversible.

TRANSPORT

From the cisternal space of the rough ER, the secretory proteins are transported into the Golgi complex. In most cells this is an organelle with distinct polarity; a receiving and packaging way station which typically consists of a series of parallel stacked smooth membrane saccules plus some associated vesicles and vacuoles. The stacks usually are arranged in the form of a shallow cup whose convex entry side faces the rough ER and whose concave or exit side faces the secretory pole of the cell. The intracellular transport of secretory protein in the exocrine pancreas was first analyzed by Caro and Palade (7) in autoradiographic experiments. Greater time resolution was obtained by Jamieson and Palade (8), who applied precise pulse labeling followed by effective removal (chase) of the unincorporated label.

Their pulse-chase experiments revealed that the secretory proteins from their site of synthesis move into the so-called transitional elements, which are portions of the ER that are devoid of ribosomes. What appeared to occur next is that these transitional elements of the ER bud off small transporting vesicles, which act as carriers for secretory protein between ER and Golgi. As soon as seven minutes after the pulse, considerable "activity" was found in the peripheral Golgi vesicles, which subsequently moved to the condensing vacuoles and the zymogen granules (see Fig. 4). According to these authors the connection between ER and Golgi is intermittent and established by shuttling vesicles. According to other investigators, however, the two compartments are permanently interconnected. For example, in the liver permanent tubular interconnections seem to exist between rough ER and Golgi system.

The process of transport from ER to Golgi appears to be independent from protein synthesis itself. After application of cycloheximide, which arrests protein synthesis, the already synthesized proteins continue to drain into the Golgi complex. However, when the cells are treated with inhibitors of respiration (cyanide) or with uncouplers of oxidative phosphorylation (dinitrophenol), the transport to the Golgi complex ceases almost immediately.

As yet, the energy requiring reactions are unknown. Recently, Locke and Huie (9) have described beadlike rings in the ER-Golgi transition zone, through which the smooth vesicles bud in order to enter the Golgi region. Perhaps these rings form the 'lock' which requires energy to open and

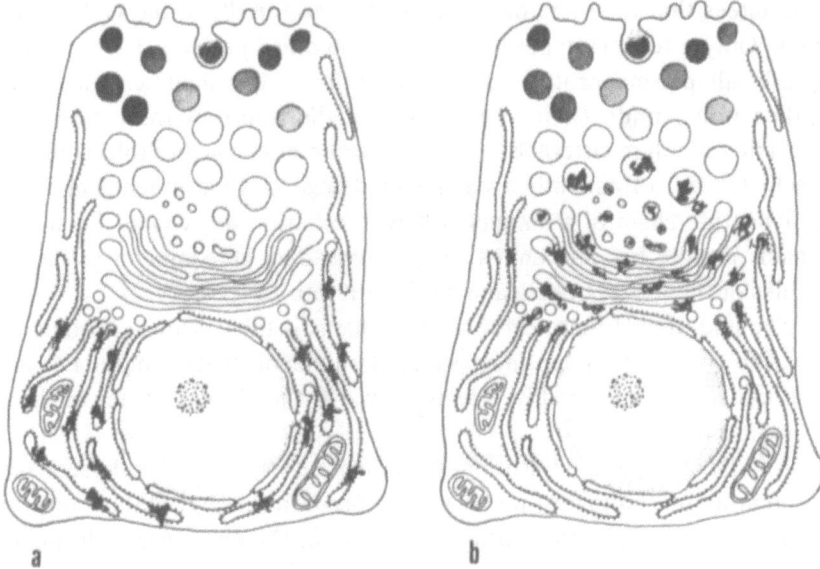

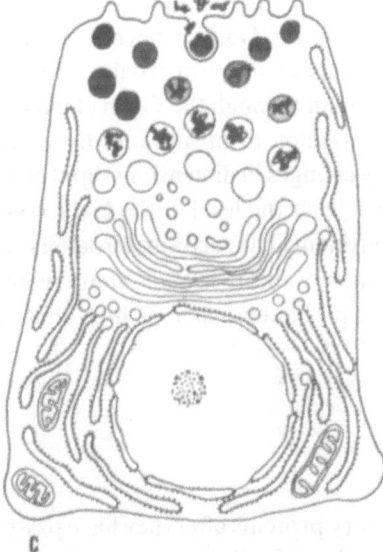

Fig. 4. Localization of radioactivity in the exocrine pancreatic cell after a short pulse labeling with ^{3}H-leucine. These grains are first present over the rER (a), then over the Golgi area (b) and subsequently over the condensing and storage granules (c). For further explanation see text. After data from 7 and 8.

guarantees that the secretory proteins flow vectorially to the Golgi complex. Only a few cell types do secrete unmodified proteins. For example, nearly all plasma proteins are glyco-proteins. The modification of the naked polypeptide chains occurs during the transport from the endoplasmic reticulum cisternae to the Golgi complex and in the Golgi complex itself. The most frequently occurring modification is the attachment to the polypeptide chain of a number of oligosaccharide side chains. Such side chains usually become linked to the asparagine, threonine or serine residues of the peptide chain and modifies it into a glycoprotein.

The addition of these carbohydrate chains is the task of a set of highly specific glycosylating enzymes, situated on the membranes of the ER and the Golgi and presumably oriented towards the cisternal space of these compartments.

Another type of modification, sometimes necessary to give the secreted protein its full biological potency, may occur in this part of the transport route. For example, the partial proteolysis of the precursor molecule of insulin (proinsulin) occurs in or close to the Golgi area of the pancreatic B-cells.

The passage of albumin through the Golgi complex has been a point of some concern because albumin is not a glycoprotein and does not need to acquire glycosyl constituents as do other plasmaproteins. According to Peters (10), there is no definite proof that the albumin is actually within the Golgi cisternae. However, in submicrosomal preparation, the albumin content parallels the concentration of typical "Golgi" enzymes such as galactosyl transferase. Perhaps the proteolytic cleavage of proalbumin into albumin is the reason for passage of albumin through the Golgi elements.

Along the export route a gradual conversion of membranes from one type to another occurs as exemplified by changes in dimensions, lipid composition and enzymatic activities. Especially at the level of the Golgi complex this membrane differentiation is pertinent. The secretory products are transferred from a highly permeable membrane to a membrane whose lipid composition approaches that of the plasmalemma in its high content of cholesterol and sphingomyelin.

CONCENTRATION AND STORAGE

Concentration and storage of the secretory proteins after they have passed the Golgi complex occurs in a great number of cell types. So for example

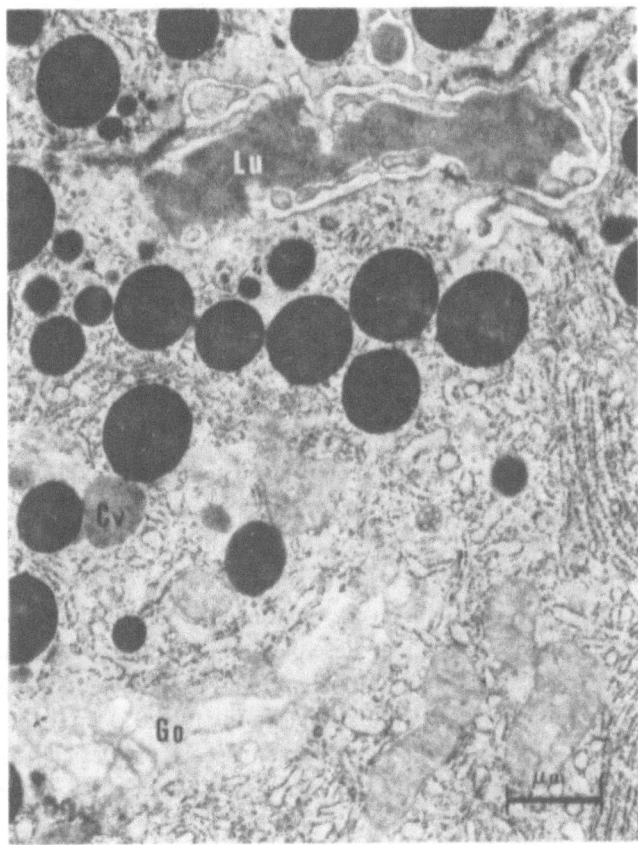

Fig. 5. Supranuclear region of exocrine pancreas cell with elements of the Golgi complex (Go), condensing vacuoles (Cv), storage vacuoles and released protein in the acinar lumen (Lu).

in both the exocrine and the endocrine cells of the pancreas. The increasing electrondensity of the secretory vacuoles in the Golgi area (Fig. 5) suggests a mechanism of concentration by removal of fluid from these condensing vacuoles. It is of importance, however, that this concentration appears to occur without the continuous supply of energy. It seems unlikely that ion pumps, located in the membranes of the condensing vacuoles, are responsible for the mechanism of concentration.

Some protein secretions are stored in vesicles in the form of complexes with metal ions (insulin with Zn^{++}, parotid amylase with Ca^{++}), presumably to facilitate storage at high concentrations. It has also been postulated that a progressive aggregation of protein molecules into "super molecules" with a consequent drop in osmotic pressure of the vacuolar content, occurs through ionic interaction between proteins of different charge or between proteins and acid mucopolysaccharides. An anionic polysulfate, presumably a sulfated peptide and probably involved in the formation of large aggregates, has recently been found in the content of pancreatic acinar secretory granules (11).

Studies on the osmotic stability of preparations of condensing vacuoles indeed suggest that the protein in zymogen granules have reduced osmotic activity. They readily lyse in alkaline solutions but their membrane can be recovered from the lysate. The mechanism of lysis at alkaline pH therefore seems to involve deaggregation of the enzymes which increases their osmotic activity.

Concentration and storage of plasma proteins within the liver is relatively insignificant, possibly because release from the cell is continuous. The 60–80 nm granules, present in the dilated bulbous ends of the Golgi saccules and in smooth vesicles between the concave Golgi face and the plasmalemma presumably are very low density lipoprotein particles (Fig. 6). It must be emphasized that these particles never appear in the central plate-like portions of the Golgi. It seems likely that there are two pathways for the extrusion of lipoprotein particles in the liver: (a) from rough ER to smooth ER elements to Golgi apparatus to secretory vesicles to plasmalemma and (b) from rough ER to smooth ER to secretory vesicles to plasmamembrane.

DISCHARGE

As a result of the sequence of events described, the cytoplasm of the secretory cell might become packed with mature vesicles, filled with material ready to be secreted. An appropriate exogenous stimulus, such as a hormone or a neurotransmitter substance is necessary to start the process of granule discharge. After approach of the secretory vesicle to the apical plasma membrane, the own membrane of the particle fuses with the plasma membrane (Fig. 7). Then an opening forms through which the content of the storage vesicle discharges into the extracellular space. This way of ejection of the secretory products is called "exocytosis" and may be regarded as the reversal of phagocytosis or pinocytosis. As in these latter events, a recognition process with a high degree of specificity is involved

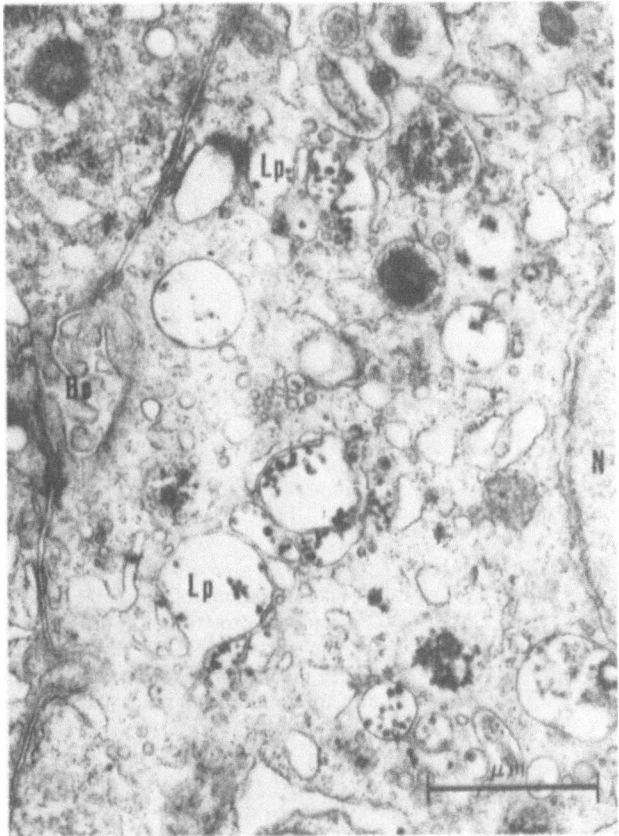

Fig. 6. Lipoprotein particles (Lp) in the Golgi vacuoles and other smooth walled vesicles in liver from a fasted rat. N = nucleus, Bc = bile capillary.

in exocytosis. For example, in the exocrine pancreas the secretory granules only fuse with the apical or luminal plasma membrane. Infrequently, a preliminary fusion of granule membrane to granule membrane occurs, so that several granules may discharge through one orifice. This type of inter-action between membranes suggests the existence of complementary re-cognition sites, possibly through specific interaction between membrane proteins, but the molecular mechanisms are unknown.

Besides a basic requirement of exocytosis for calcium ions, the actual membrane fusion and discharge are dependent on the supply of energy. ATP may serve to power the molecular reorganization of the membranes, required to fuse and then to break apart along a new plane.

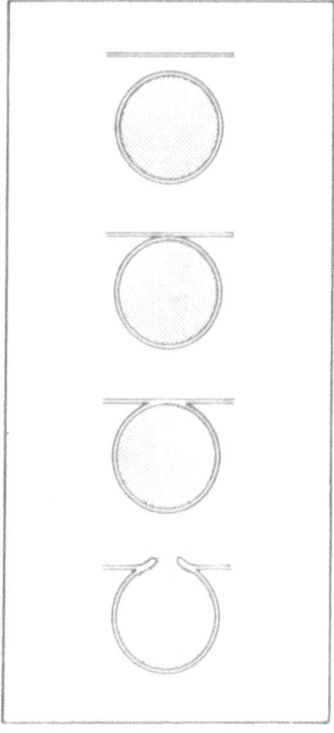

Fig. 7. Diagram of discharge of storage granules by exocytosis. The membrane of the granule first touches the plasma membrane, then the membranes merge and an opening is formed through which the proteins are released.

In many systems the actual secretory discharge is also inhibited by colchicine or cytochalasine. This suggests that microtubules and contractile microfilaments are involved, probably in directing the storage granules towards the plasma membrane.

Mainly because the secretory process requires the presence of calcium in the extracellular medium, the set of events triggered by the secretory stimulus has been called "stimulus-secretion coupling," by analogy with the "excitation-contraction coupling" which occurs in muscle cells. The biochemical events involved in the stimulus-secretion coupling are incompletely understood. A general hypothesis involves the interaction of the secretagogue with a specific receptor site on the external surface of the cell membrane. A cyclic nucleotide generating system (in most cases the enzyme adenylate cyclase) on the internal surface of the membrane is capable of converting ATP to cyclic AMP. The action of a large number of hormones has been shown to be mediated by alterations in tissue concentrations of this compound. A transducer mechanism situated between the receptor site and the catalytic site activates the enzyme in response to the binding of the hormone or neurotransmitter.

The consequence of exocytosis not only is the discharge of the secretory products, but also the insertion of the secretory granule membrane in the plasmalemma at the participating region of the cell surface. Yet the latter does not expand permanently, indicating that the cell has a mechanism for elimination of the extra material, probably by an inward budding of membrane vesicles from the plasma membrane.

In fact, the process of secretion not only involves the transport of the secretory proteins, but also of their membranous containers. It seems likely that there is a constant flow of membrane material through the cell in the secretory cycle, involving the renewal of membranes of the secretory pathway again and again. Whether the membranes are recycled for the main part or are newly synthesized after previous demolition into its constituents as part of a normal repair or turnover process, is largely unknown. In any way, the particular characteristics of each membranous component along the intracellular secretory pathway must remain intact, in order to guarantee the continuous functioning of the cell.

REFERENCES

1. Palade GE: Intracellular aspects of the process of protein synthesis. Science 189:347–358, 1975.
2. Andrews TM, Tata JR: Protein synthesis by membrane-bound and free ribosomes of secretory and non-secretory tissues. Biochem J 121:683–694, 1971.
3. Lin C, Chang J: Electron microscopy of albumin synthesis. Science 190:465–467, 1975.
4. Sabatini DD, Blobel G: Controlled proteolysis of nascent polypeptides in rat liver cell fractions. II Location of the polypeptides in rough microsomes. J Cell Biol 45:146–157, 1970.
5. Adelman MR, Sabatini DD, Blobel G: Ribosome membrane interaction. Non-destructive disassembly of rat liver rough microsomes into ribosomal and membranous components. J Cell Biol 56:206–239, 1973.
6. Blobel G, Sabatini DD: Ribosome-membrane interaction in eukaryotic cells. Biomembranes 2:193–195, 1973.
7. Caro LG, Palade GE: Protein synthesis, storage and discharge in the pancreatic exocrine cell. An autoradiographic study. J Cell Biol 20:473–495, 1964.
8. Jamieson JD, Palade GE: Intracellular transport of secretory proteins in the pancreatic exocrine cell. I. Role of the peripheral elements of the Golgi complex. J Cell Biol 34:577–596, 1967.
9. Locke M, Huie P: Golgi complex-endoplasmic reticulum transition region has rings of beads. Science 188:1219–1220, 1975.

10. Peters T: Cellular protein transport. In: Albumin and Abnormal Protein Biosynthesis, MA Rothschild, M Oratz, SS Schreiber (eds), New York, Pergamon Press, 1975, pp 111–136.
11. Tartakoff A, Greene LJ, Palade GE: Studies on the guinea pig pancreas. Fractionation and partial characterization of exocrine proteins. J Biol Chem 249:7420–7431, 1974.

3. Molecular approach to the study of albumin synthesis

D.A. Shafritz, R.K. Strair, and S.H. Yap

Although serum albumin was originally recognized and described by Ancell as early as 1837 (1), it has only been possible to obtain insight into the mechanism for albumin synthesis in the past 10–15 years. The purpose of this chapter is to describe methods developed recently to study albumin synthesis at the molecular level. However, since classical methods still have more clinical relevance, we would like to mention briefly some of these approaches. Initial studies were devoted to the simple measurement of serum albumin levels in normal individuals and patients with various disorders and Dr. Majoor made a number of significant contributions in this area (2). Subsequently, a variety of radioactive labeling procedures were developed which permitted determination of the serum half-life ($T_{1/2}$) for this protein (3). This involved intravenous injection of tracer doses of radioactive labeled albumin into patients with hypoalbuminenia and determination of the radioactive decay curve for injected material. Assuming that synthesis of albumin is equivalent to its rate of loss or degradation and that the serum pool is at steady state, a rate for albumin synthesis can be calculated indirectly from the serum decay curve (4). The next major advance in studying albumin synthesis was the development by McFarlane and colleagues of a method to measure albumin synthesis rate directly in whole animals. As these investigators recognized, there was a direct correlation between incorporation of arginine into albumin and urea synthesis, and measurement of labelled arginine in albumin after injection of ^{14}C carbonate versus urea production could be used to calculate albumin synthesis (5). Techniques were then advanced to permit studies of albumin synthesis in the isolated – perfused liver (6), and this model has provided us with much useful information on factors involved in the regulation of albumin synthesis. These topics will be explored in depth in subsequent chapters.

Studies on hepatic synthesis and secretion of albumin at the molecular level began in the 1960's, and knowledge in this area has advanced rapidly during the past decade. Our initial studies were prompted by the observation that the synthesis of secretory proteins, such as albumin, occurred primarily on membrane-bound polyribosomes, whereas synthesis of cytosol proteins, such as ferritin, occurred primarily on free polyribosomes (7). The mechanism for this apparent segregation of albumin synthesizing polyribosomes (and presumably albumin mRNA) represented to us a fascinating aspect of subcellular control. A great deal of information has also been gathered on the mechanism for synthesis of secretory proteins as precursor molecules. This has led to the proposal of a generalized model for synthesis of secretory proteins, which will be presented later. Specific evidence for synthesis of albumin as a precursor has been obtained and the possible role of this precursor in subcellular compartmentalization of albumin synthesizing polyribosomes and albumin secretion will be discussed. Data to suggest that alterations in some of these processes may occur in experimental models for certain pathologic disorders will be presented in chapter 4.

PREPARATION OF LIVER POLYRIBOSOMES AND CELL-FREE PROTEIN SYNTHESIS

To examine synthesis of albumin at the molecular level, we initially prepared membrane-bound and free polyribosomes from rabbit liver by a combination of the procedures of Blobel and Potter (8) and Bloemendal et al. (9). This consisted essentially of homogenizing liver in a buffered solution of 0.25 M sucrose, preparing a post-mitochondrial supernatant fraction (material soluble after centrifugation at $17,300 \times g$ for 10 min.) and separating membrane-bound from free polyribosomes by high speed centrifugation ($131,000 \times g$ for 8 hrs.) through a two-layer discontinuous sucrose gradient (7). As shown schematically in Fig. 1, supernatant protein remains in the 0.25 M sucrose zone of the gradient. Free polyribosomes sediment through 1.8 M sucrose to the bottom of the tube, whereas intact membrane-bound polyribosomes collect at the interface between 1.45 M and 1.8 M sucrose. Membranes devoid of ribosomes (or containing very few ribosomes) migrate to the interface between 0.25 M and 1.45 M sucrose. The polyribosomes fractions are withdrawn by aspiration and recentrifuged through a second discontinuous gradient to increase their purity.

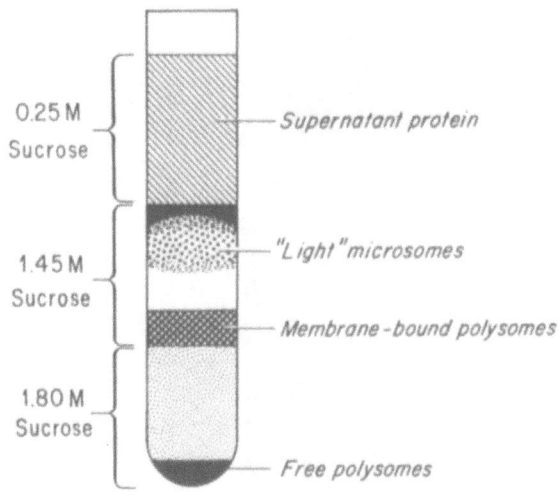

Fig. 1. Separation of membrane-bound and free polyribosomes by discontinuous sucrose gradient centrifugation.

Rabbit liver 105,000 × g supernatant protein is included in each gradient layer as a ribonuclease inhibitor. Heparin is also present in the original cellular homogenization buffer. Fig. 2 shows the transmission electron-microscopic appearance of purified membrane-bound and free polyribosomes after the second discontinuous gradient, as well as the appearance of the non polysome-containing membrane fraction. More recently, we have utilized the procedure of Ramsey and Steele (10) to prepare membrane-bound and free polyribosomes, and this procedure provides quantitative yields of both fractions with high activity in cell-free protein synthesis (10, 11). Crude membrane-bound polysomes are first separated (together with nuclei, mitochondria, and other particulate components) from free liver polyribosomes by centrifugation at 131,000 × g for 12 min. Membrane-bound polyribosomes are then separated from nuclei by centrifugation at 1470 × g for 5 min. and the membranes are subsequently lysed by addition of sodium deoxycholate. Polyribosomes are collected by discontinuous sucrose gradient centrifugation (rat liver supernatant is included as a ribonuclease inhibitor). The sucrose gradient distribution profiles of membrane-bound and free liver polyribosomes obtained by this procedure are shown in Fig. 3. There is good preservation of polyribosome size in animals fed a normal diet, although free polyribosomes generally show a

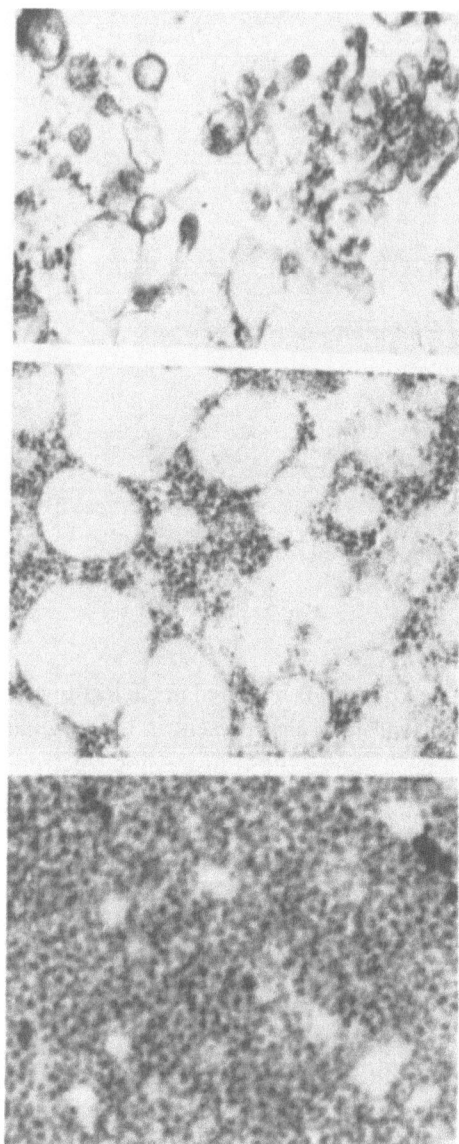

Fig. 2. Appearance of membrane-bound and free liver polyribosomes on transmission electron microscopy. Upper frame, smooth membranes; middle frame membrane-found polyribosomes; lower frame, free polyribosomes.

slightly larger average size then membrane-bound polyribosomes (this is probably due to residual ribonuclease activity in the membrane fraction or possibly other technical reasons). However, in animals fasted for

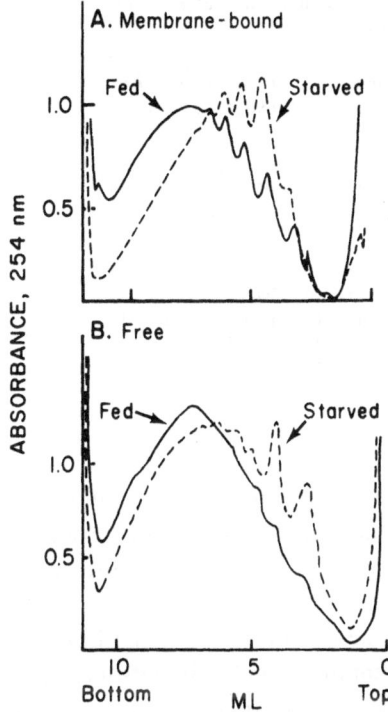

Fig. 3. Distribution profile on continuous sucrose gradient centrifugation of membrane-bound and free liver polyribosomes from fed versus fasted rats. A. Membrane-bound polyribosomes, B. Free polyribosomes.

24–30 hrs. prior to sacrifice, there is considerable disaggregation of membrane-bound polyribosomes. We have also noted a generalized decrease in cell-free protein synthesis activity of polyribosomes obtained from fasted animals, and similar observations have been made by other investigators (6, 12, 13). Our results on the direct measurement of albumin mRNA under these conditions will be given in chapter 4.

The question we wished to approach was whether there is an actual segregation of albumin mRNA in membrane-bound versus free polyribosomes, or whether the differences observed by previous investigators are the result of translation or post-translational control events. For this purpose we initially employed the technique of in vitro protein synthesis coupled with a characterization of albumin in the cell-free reaction product by both immunological and chemical repurification (7). As shown in Table 1 when the data are expressed as the % of total protein synthesis representing albumin, there is a clear distinction between membrane-bound and free liver polyribosomes. Regardless of whether, total immuno-logically reactive material or chemically repurified protein (electrophoretic

Table 1. Albumin synthesis by membrane-bound and free liver polysomes versus their respective mRNA extracts

Polysomes	Liver system endogenous mRNA	Reticulocyte system exogenous mRNA
	Immunological Precipitation (albumin % total protein synthesis)	
Free	0.89	0.96
Membrane-bound	5.0	1.13
	Chemical Repurification (albumin % total protein synthesis)	
Free	0.20	1.17
Membrane-bound	1.74	0.95

and size characteristics of albumin) is monitored, membrane-bound polyribosomes synthesized 5–8 times more albumin than free polyribosomes.
The same interpretation could be reached when the data are expressed as
albumin synthesis per μg liver polysomal RNA (data not shown). Since the
traditional method for isolating membrane-bound and free polyribosomes
gave unpredictable, low yields for membrane-bound polyribosomes, and
since more of the albumin mRNA in the cytoplasm might not be present in
polyribosomes, we were unable to estimate the total subcellular distribution of albumin synthesizing activity. However, it was clear from these
results as well as other studies (14–17) that we were effectively able to
separate membrane-bound from free polyribosomes and that commonly
employed methods permitted us to distinguish albumin synthesis in these
fractions.

As mentioned earlier, the above data and many other findings suggested
that membrane-bound and free polyribosomes synthesize different classes
of proteins and that there is mRNA segregation within various subcellular compartments (7, 14–17). These conclusions were based on the
assumption that each mRNA in a given ribosomal population is translated
with a constant relative efficiency at all times. Unfortunately, few data were
available to confirm this assumption and it was also possible that other
mechanisms might contribute to regulation of specific protein synthesis in
membrane-bound versus free polyribosomes. To begin an evaluation of
this problem, we extracted total RNA from liver membrane-bound and
free polyribosomes and translated this RNA in a heterologous, fractionated
reticulocyte cell-free system. The use of a heterologous system (i.e.

ribosomes from another cell type, which did not normally synthesize the protein in question) ensured that specific synthesis of albumin would truly represent addition of exogenous RNA and not simply stimulation of endogenous mRNA translation (18). This same method was used in the original studies demonstrating isolation and translation of globin mRNA by Lingrel and coworkers (19). Our reticulocyte system was separately dependent on added ribosomes, supernatant factors, initiation factors and mRNA, and we hoped that this system would enable us to study the mechanism for albumin synthesis, as well as various aspects of subcellular control. When RNA fractions from the same preparations of membrane-bound versus free liver polyribosomes as used previously were translated in the reticulocyte cell-free system (Table 1), there was little difference between the two RNA preparations in the percentage synthesis of albumin. These results were rather surprising and suggested several possibilities: 1) that there was little difference in the level of albumin mRNA in these preparations and that non-translated albumin mRNA was present in free polyribosomes [this mRNA could be present as contaminating mRNA-protein complexes (mRNPs)]; 2) that features other than mRNA, such as initiation or other specific protein synthesis factors controlled translation in membrane-bound versus free polyribosomes; or 3) that the level of specific mRNA translation in a heterologous cell-free system did not necessarily reflect the level of that specific mRNA in the total RNA preparation. The first and third hypotheses have been evaluated extensively in our laboratory during the past 2–3 years; however, since protein synthesis in the membrane system is rather complex and the amount of protein synthesis factors which can be obtained from membrane-bound polyribosomes rather limited, we have not been able to evaluate directly to the second possibility.

USE OF MOLECULAR HYBRIDIZATION TO ISOLATE, QUANTITATE AND STUDY THE METABOLISM OF ALBUMIN mRNA

As mentioned above, a variety of difficulties may be encountered when protein synthesis is used to quantitate the level of a specific mRNA in a given polyribosome preparation. Originally, we had hoped that translation of exogenous mRNA in a heterologous system, with rigorous identification of specific product, would permit us to make such measurements. However, it soon became evident that these methods would fall short of our intended goal, since other investigators reported that many factors, such as 1) the cell-free system used for translation (20), 2) the concentration of mono-valent and divalent cations (21, 22), 3) the presence of hemin, polyamines and other activators or inhibitors of protein synthesis (23–30), 4) the nature of the mRNA under investigation (20), 5) the use of purified versus mixed preparations of mRNA (31–35), and 6) the level of certain initiation factors in the system, primarily IF-M_3 and/or IF-M_4 (36–38), may influence trans-lation of a given mRNA. Therefore, we felt it was essential to find an alternative, more direct assay for specific mRNA. In the early 1970's, Temin and Mizutani (39) and Baltimore (40) reported the isolation of an enzyme capable of synthesizing DNA from mRNA in a cell-free system. For this discovery Temin and Baltimore shared the Nobel Prize in Physio-logy and Medicine in 1975. The enzyme, referred to as "reverse transcript-ase", requires only an RNA template containing a 3'-poly (A) sequence, oligo $(dT)_{8-12}$ primer, divalent cation (Mg^{++}), actinomycin D (to prevent synthesis of DNA-DNA hybrids), and all four deoxyribonucleoside tri-phosphates (d XTP's) (Fig. 4). Due to Watson-Crick base-pairing, DNA synthesized from mRNA is complementary in base sequence (referred to as cDNA) and after synthesis is linked by hydrogen-bonds to the mRNA template. mRNA can be digested from the hybrids by addition of alkali and the cDNA collected by ETOH precipitation and/or sucrose gradient

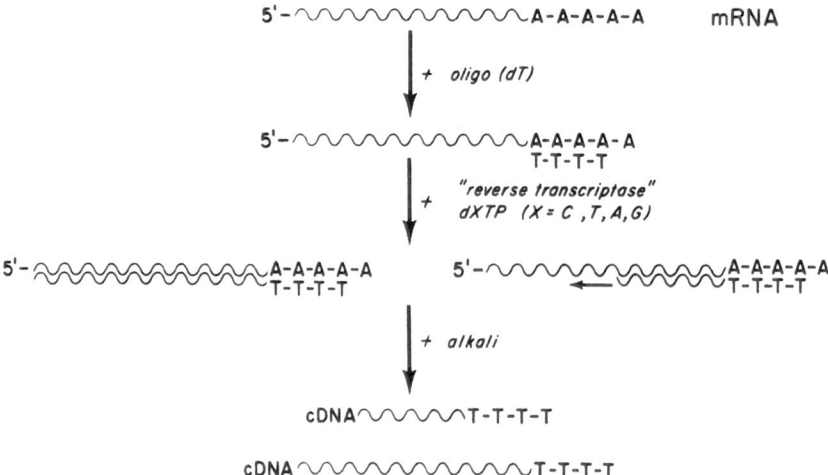

Fig. 4. Synthesis of complementary DNA (cDNA) from mRNA by the use of "reverse transcriptase."

centrifugation. Using high specific activity dXTP substrates, the cDNA can be labeled to very high specific activity (20×10^6 cpm/μg). Under appropriate annealing conditions, this material can be used as an accurate and highly sensitive probe for detecting RNA sequences to which the cDNA is specifically complementary. This assay is ~ 1000 times more sensitive for mRNA than the most sensitive protein synthesizing system, the frog oocyte (20). One potential limitation, however, should be mentioned; namely, that the mRNA need not be intact or biologically active to hybridize with cDNA.

The actual assay for analytical molecular hybridization is shown schematically in Fig. 5. An RNA sample is mixed with labeled cDNA in

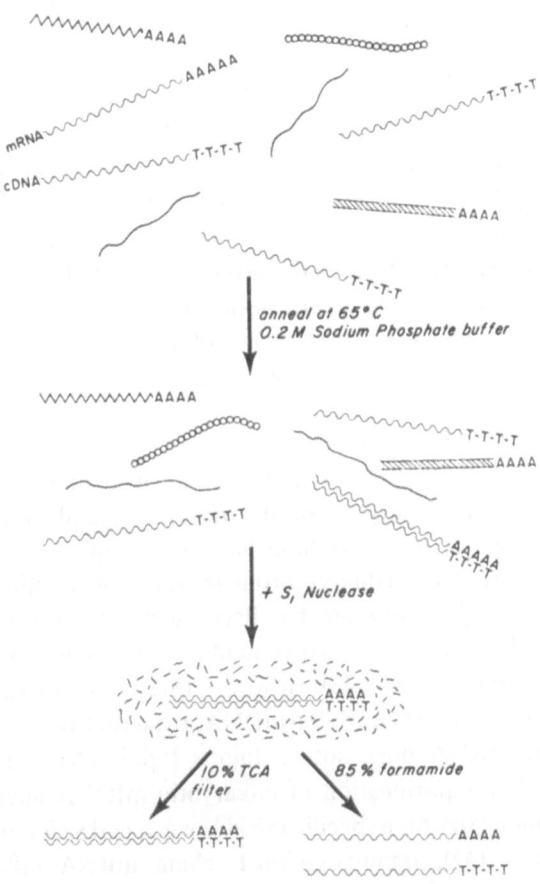

Fig. 5. Molecular hybridization assay for quantitation of messenger RNA.

phosphate buffer and other reaction components. The material is drawn up into a capillary tube, which is sealed, boiled at 100°C and incubated at elevated temperature under conditions in which only sequences which are fully complementary will form hybrids (stringent conditions). After the appropriate incubation period, which depends on the type of analysis being performed, material is expelled from the capillary tube into a solution containing S_1 nuclease. This nuclease, isolated from *Aspergillus oryzae*, will digest all remaining single stranded sequences or molecules, leaving intact only mRNA-cDNA hybrids. These hybrids are precipitated with trichloroacetic acid in the cold and collected on nitrocellulose filters for counting by liquid scintillation spectroscopy. For most of our experiments, RNA excess hybridization has been employed (41, 42). In simple terms, hybrid formation is a bimolecular reaction following second order kinetics. However, when RNA is present in large excess compared to DNA, the reaction follows pseudo first order kinetics and the rate of hybrid formation depends only on the initial concentration of RNA and the time period of incubation. The term Rot (mol.-sec./1) is the product of Ro (concentration of RNA at time 0) and t (incubation time), and the percentage of cDNA hybridized is a function of these two variables. For a specific mRNA component, the $Rot_{1/2}$ is the product of initial RNA concentration and time required to hybridize 50% of the cDNA input. When this value is compared to a known RNA standard of given molecular weight, the sequence complexity (total mass of unique polyribonucleotide sequences in the RNA preparation) can be calculated. For a mathematical treatment of hybridization analysis see ref. 43.

In order to use hybridization analysis to measure albumin mRNA content, it was first necessary to purify the mRNA and prepare albumin ^{3}H-cDNA probe. Various procedures have been employed for purification of eukaryotic mRNAs. Affinity chromatography with either oligo (dT)-cellulose or poly (U)-sepharose has been most successful for separating mRNAs containing a 3'-poly (A) segment from the bulk of ribosomal and other RNA components (44, 45). However, this procedure cannot be used to separate specific polyadenylated mRNAs from each other, and a portion of eukaryotic mRNA does not contain a 3'-poly (A) segment (46, 47). Other methods for purification of eukaryotic mRNAs have been based either on a unique size for a specific mRNA, e.g. α and β globin mRNA (19), histone mRNA (47), immunoglobin-L chain mRNA (48), ovalbumin mRNA (49), etc; or an unusual nucleotide composition, e.g. silk fibroin mRNA (50). Commonly used procedures for separation of RNA molecules according to size (e.g. sucrose gradient centrifugation and gel electrophoresis) have been successful only for mRNAs which represent a large proportion of total cellular mRNA, such as globin mRNA in reticulocytes, ovalbumin mRNA in the estrogen stimulated chick oviduct, or immunoglobulin mRNA in myeloma cells. Another method which has given excellent results is hybridization of total RNA to a specific DNA-cellulose affinity column (51), but this procedure again requires initial purification of the mRNA by traditional methods in order to generate the cDNA-cellulose.

For purification of mRNAs which are average sized and are present as only a small portion of total cellular mRNA, the method of immunoprecipitation of polysomes containing nascent polypeptide chains for a specific protein is the only specific procedure available at the present time. Immunoprecipitation can enrich a polysome preparation for a specific mRNA by 5–10 fold (52, 53). However, in order to obtain intact mRNA with good biological activity, the antibody must be highly purified to remove ribonuclease activity. Furthermore, large amounts of antibody are needed to generate sufficient amounts of material for use in molecular studies. In our investigations, we have combined the techniques of immunoprecipitation of albumin specific polyribosomes and controlled molecular hybridization in a novel approach to prepare highly purified rat albumin mRNA. The general strategy of our procedure is to first enrich for a specific mRNA, so that it represents the most abundant sequence in a given RNA population. Complementary DNA is transcribed from this enriched mRNA and is then used in a limited RNA-cDNA hybridization, under conditions in which only cDNA corresponding to the most abundant component of the RNA population from which it was transcribed, will form hybrids (selection of the appropriate Rot). In practical term, a large excess of RNA is used and the incubation time is adjusted so that only 10% of the most frequent component will form hybrids. Although this approach sacrifices yield, a highly purified RNA can be obtained. Messenger RNA is then isolated from the RNA-cDNA hybrid and the controlled hybridization procedure can be repeated, if necessary. The mRNA is characterized for purity by molecular hybridization and cell-free protein synthesis. By these procedures we have prepared biologically active, highly purified, rat albumin mRNA and an albumin cDNA probe which can be utilized for a variety of molecular studies.

Fig. 6 shows schematically the purification procedure as we have adapted it for large scale purification of rat albumin mRNA. Liver polyribosomes

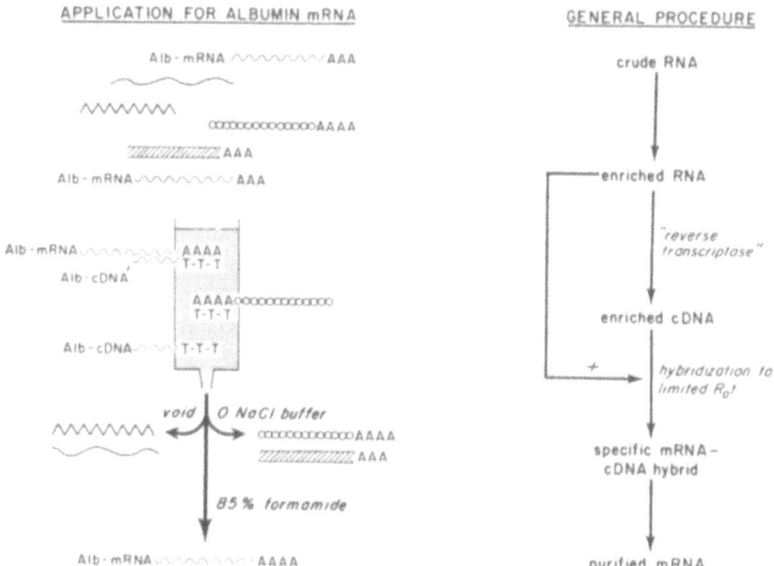

Fig. 6. Purification of albumin mRNA by controlled molecular hybridization on albumin cDNA cellulose.

containing nascent chains for albumin are selected from total deoxycholate treated polyribosomes by indirect immunoprecipitation, producing a sub-fraction of albumin mRNA enriched polyribosomes (41). RNA is prepared from these polyribosomes by phenol:chloroform:isoamyl alcohol (50:48: 2v/v) extraction and poly A containing mRNA isolated by oligo (dT)-cellu-lose chromatography. cDNA directly linked to cellulose is then prepared from the albumin mRNA enriched fraction by incubation of the mRNA template directly with oligo (dT)-cellulose primer in the presence of "reverse transcriptase". The mRNA is digested from the cellulose by treatment with alkali and cDNA enriched for albumin mRNA sequences remains cova-lently linked to the oligo (dT)-cellulose. This material is then used for con-trolled hybridization (hybridization to a limited Rot) with a separate ali-quot of either albumin mRNA enriched RNA or crude liver poly A$^+$ RNA. The mRNA-cDNA cellulose hybrid is placed in a column and unadsorbed material, as well as material forming hybrids in only the poly (A)-oligo(dT) region, are removed from the cellulose by successive washings with column buffer and salt free buffer, respectively. Specific albumin mRNA is eluted from the column with 85% (v/v) formamide (an effective denaturing agent which disrupts hydrogen-bond base pairs between mRNA and cDNA), and this material can be subsequently isolated and used for hybridization studies and cell-free protein synthesis. Figs. 7, 8, 9 show the hybridization analysis of the various RNA and cDNA fractions obtained by this procedure. Crude total poly A$^+$ liver mRNA was hybridized to cDNA prepared from itself, and as can be seen in Fig. 7, there is no obvious component which hybridizes rapidly and represents a significant portion of total cDNA. However, it would be difficult to recognize such a component unless it represented at least 10% of total liver cytoplasmic poly A$^+$ RNA. In fact, there is the suggestion of a specific component in the 5–10% range. With cDNA prepared from albumin immunoprecipitated polyribosomes approximately 30% of the material hybridizes as a single complexity component with either crude poly A$^+$ RNA or immunoprecipitation enriched cDNA (Fig. 8). When cDNA is prepared from the highly purified mRNA fraction eluted from albumin cDNA-cellulose, this cDNA fraction hybridizes to 80–85% with either crude total poly A$^+$ RNA or immunoprecipitated poly A$^+$ RNA (Fig. 9). It should also be noted that the hybridization analyses of crude, partially purified, or highly purified material all show a specific complexity component with a log $Rot_{1/2}$ between -2 and -3. Further characterization of the highly purified mRNA fraction will be presented in Chapter 4.

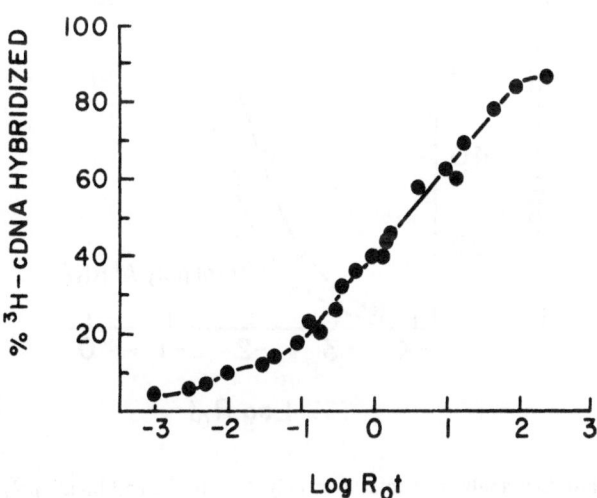

Fig. 7. Hybridization analysis of total liver poly A$^+$ mRNA with total liver cDNA.

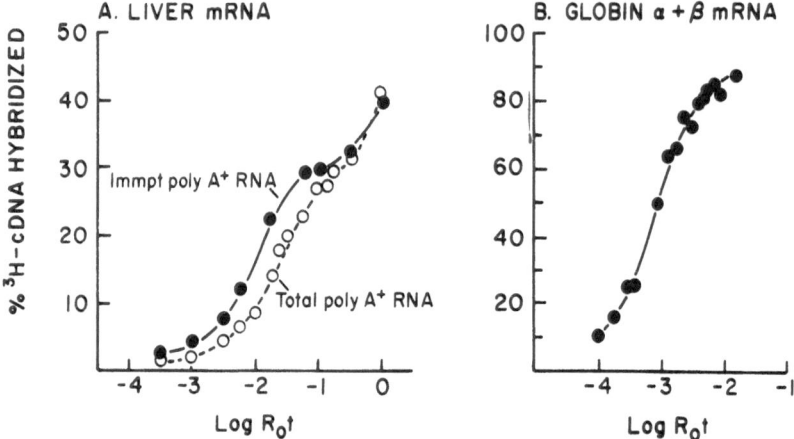

Fig. 8. Hybridization analysis of total liver poly A$^+$ mRNA and poly A$^+$ mRNA from polyribosomes immunoprecipitated with albumin antibody (Immpt poly A$^+$ RNA). In these experiments the ^{3}H-cDNA utilized was prepared from Immpt poly. A$^+$ mRNA.

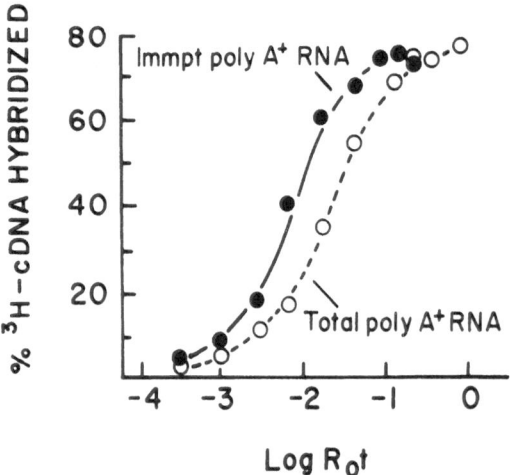

Fig. 9. Hybridization analysis of total liver poly A$^+$ mRNA and Immpt poly A$^+$ mRNA with purified albumin ^{3}H-cDNA.

MECHANISM FOR SYNTHESIS OF SECRETORY PROTEINS

During the past few years considerable progress has been made on the general mechanism for synthesis of secretory proteins, and two basic models have emerged (Fig. 10). According to the first model (Fig. 10A) advanced by Blobel and coworkers (54, 55), formation of polyribosomes and translation of mRNA for all proteins begins in the cytosol compartment of the cell. Those mRNAs whose translation products are to be transferred across a membrane first synthesize a hydrophobic N-terminal

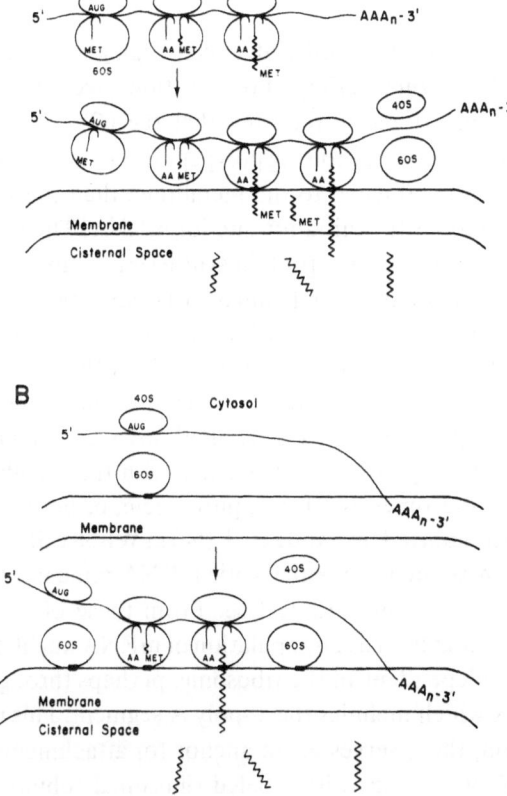

Fig. 10. Schematic representation of general mechanisms proposed for synthesis of secretory proteins in animal cells.

peptide, which serves as the signal for recognition by the membrane. Polyribosomes containing this hydrophobic peptide or "signal sequence" attach to the membrane and polypeptide synthesis continues. The N-terminal peptide is cleaved by a specific enzyme residing in the membrane, so that it does not appear in the final product. Once the protein has entered the membrane, synthesis continues vectorially through the membrane and the completed product is released into the intra-cisternal space. Details concerning specific steps in this mechanism are less well established, but the model has many attractive features. Results from our own studies with vescicular stomatitis virus (VSV)-infected HeLa cells, in which case we could follow the entry into the membrane of labeled glycoprotein GmRNA (an mRNA specific for the membrane fraction), are consistent with this model (56), as are several other recent reports (57–59).

An alternative model (Fig. 10B), advanced originally by Sabatini and co-workers (60), is based on a variety of observations over the past ten years. Originally, these investigators reported that the 60S ribosomal subunit, which carries the nascent or growing polypeptide chain during protein synthesis, is more firmly attached to the membrane than the 40S ribosomal subunit, which contains the initiation site for mRNA. The 60S subunit can also attach to membranes when protein synthesis is inhibited by cycloheximide or cmetine. Rosbash and Penman (61) have defined two specific subcategories of membrane-bound ribosomes in HeLa cells ("loose" and "tight"). Other investigators have reported in liver that albumin synthesis occurs specifically on tightly bound ribosomes (62). Subsequently Milcarek and Penman (63) observed that a portion of mRNA in membrane-bound polyribosomes is tightly bound and remains with the membrane fraction after removal of ribosomes by EDTA, puromycin, or both agents. Similar results have been reported by Lande et al. (64) in WI-38 cells, and it appears that the 3'-poly A sequence of eukaryotic mRNA remains attached to the membrane after treatment with RNase. From these observations it has been proposed that at least a subpopulation of mRNA might be attached to the membrane independent of the ribosome, perhaps through an mRNA-protein complex which includes the 3'-poly A segment. This mRNA-membrane interaction, then, serves as an anchor for attachment of ribosomal subunits. Based on findings with labeled ribosomal subunits and labeled initiator tRNA, a similar model has been proposed in myeloma cells by Mechler and Vasalli (65).

EVIDENCE FOR SYNTHESIS OF ALBUMIN AS A PRECURSOR MOLECULE

The "signal sequence" hypothesis (Blobel and coworkers) predicts that serum albumin is synthesized in the liver as a precursor molecule. Evidence for such a precursor has been obtained by several investigators. During attempts to purify labeled albumin from rat liver extracts, Judah and Nicholls (66, 67) noted that immunoprecipitation with a specific albumin antibody yielded a product contaminated by a highly labeled "impurity." The "impurity" was not present in rat serum albumin and was separated from liver albumin by DEAE cellulose chromatography. They suggested that this "impurity" represented a polypeptide precursor to serum albumin (66, 67). On limited tryptic hydrolysis, the precursor yielded a peptide fragment of ~ 600 daltons not obtained with purified serum albumin (68). Similar studies by Russel and Geller (69) demonstrated an "albumin-like" protein which was separated from serum albumin by isoelectric focusing. The "albumin-like" protein was highly labeled and differed in isoelectric point from serum albumin by 0.24 pH units. Tryptic peptide mapping of the labeled "albumin-like" protein yielded a pattern identical to serum albumin, except for one additional peptide spot (70). In total liver (71), in single liver cells in suspension (72), and in certain hepatomas (73), Schreiber and co-workers have also identified an albumin precursor molecule containing an extra N-terminal oligopeptide. This oligopeptide consists of 5–6 amino acids and has been sequenced by Russel and Geller (70) as (arg)-gly-val-phe-arg-arg and by Urban et al. (71) as gly-val-phe-ser-arg. These results are consistent with the synthesis of albumin as a precursor molecule, but the precursor identified by these investigators is shorter than that predicted from the "signal hypothesis." This polypeptide segment is also hydrophilic in character, rather than hydrophobic, and the molecule is generally referred to as proalbumin. The ratio of proalbumin to albumin is highest in the rough endoplasmic reticulum, intermediate in the Golgi apparatus and lowest in the smooth endoplasmic reticulum (74). Proalbumin has also been isolated from human liver (75).

Evidence for synthesis of preproalbumin (with a hydrophobic precursor segment) has recently been obtained by Strauss et al. (76). This protein was synthesized in a wheat germ cell-free system under direction of crude rat liver mRNA. Labeled albumin was isolated from the cell-free reaction product by immunoprecipitation and SDS-polyacrylamide gel electrophoresis and the N-terminal region was analyzed by automated amino acid sequencing and compared to the known sequence of proalbumin. Wheat germ is particularly suited for synthesizing precursor proteins, since polypeptide processing does not occur in this system (57, 78). The exact relationship between preproalbumin, proalbumin and albumin is shown schematically in Fig. 11. Preproalbumin is a precursor to serum albumin containing an extra N-terminal peptide of 24 amino acids. The first 18 of these amino acids are cleaved, leaving a shorter precursor containing 5–6 amino acids, called proalbumin. This molecule is subsequently modified to the final form of albumin as found in the serum.

Combining the various data from in vivo and in vitro studies, a generalized model for synthesis and secretion of albumin can be proposed (Fig. 12). According to this model, albumin mRNA is released from the nucleus and associates with ribosomal subunits in the cytosol to form an initiation complex, as described in Chapter 4. Synthesis of the N-terminal

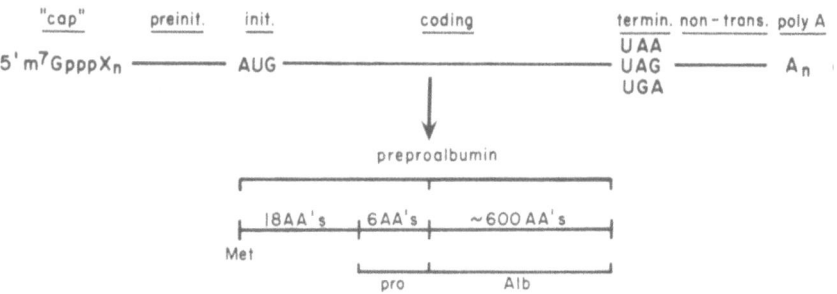

Fig. 11. Schematic diagram for the relationship between preproalbumin, proalbumin and albumin.

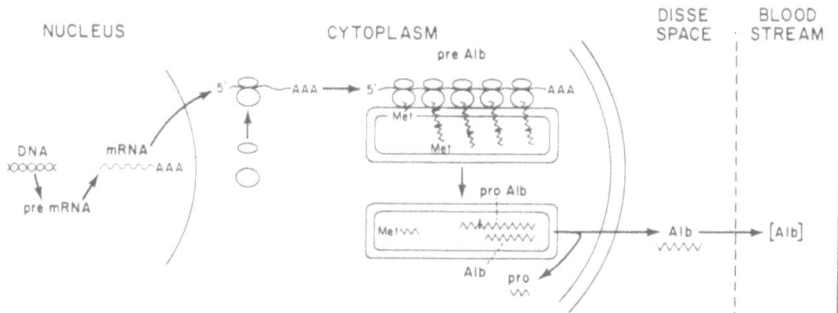

Fig. 12. Diagromatic model for the synthesis and secretion of albumin from the liver.

peptide from the coding region of the mRNA begins and a free oligosome is formed. Polypeptide synthesis continues and the nascent chain, which is hydrophobic in character, emerges through the surface of the 60S ribosomal subunit. This hydrophobic peptide interacts with hydrophobic constituents within the membrane and the polyribosome, which is becoming progressively larger, attaches to the membrane. Protein synthesis continues and most of the N-terminal precursor segment is cleaved by a peptidase while the protein is still contained within the membrane. This event probably occurs before protein synthesis is completed. The N-terminal region of the protein now contains a short hydrophilic precursor segment, which may help to repel this protein from the membrane into the intracisternal space. Regardless of the exact details for this process, a vectoral synthesis of albumin across the membrane occurs and protein synthesis is completed. The short oligopeptide region is cleaved within the intracisternal space as the albumin is transported from RER to SER to secretory vacuoles. The exact nature of these processes and the final mechanism for transfer of albumin to Disse Space and to the blood stream have not been elucidated.

POTENTIAL FUTURE STUDIES ON ALBUMIN GENE EXPRESSION

Hybridization analysis can also be used to identify precursors to albumin mRNA in the nucleus. Previously, we reported in an avian reticulocyte system that globin mRNA is present in the nucleus in two precursors of larger sedimentation value than cytoplasmic globin mRNA (77). We also studied the half-life of these molecules and obtained evidence that they represent precursors to cytoplasmic globin mRNA. In the rat liver system, we have obtained evidence for a higher molecular weight precursor to albumin mRNA. When nuclear RNA is isolated from liver cells under appropriate conditions to prevent degradation, and the RNA fraction is sedimented in a sucrose gradient under conditions preventing formation of RNA-RNA aggregates, albumin mRNA sequences can be found at both 17S (the same position as cytoplasmic albumin mRNA) and 26S (Fig. 13). The latter molecules are polyadenylated and are approximately twice the size of albumin mRNA in the cytoplasm. Whether there is a kinetic relationship between the 26S and 17S molecules, as we have found with globin mRNA (77), remains to be determined. We also would like to use the hybridization techniques to measure rates of albumin

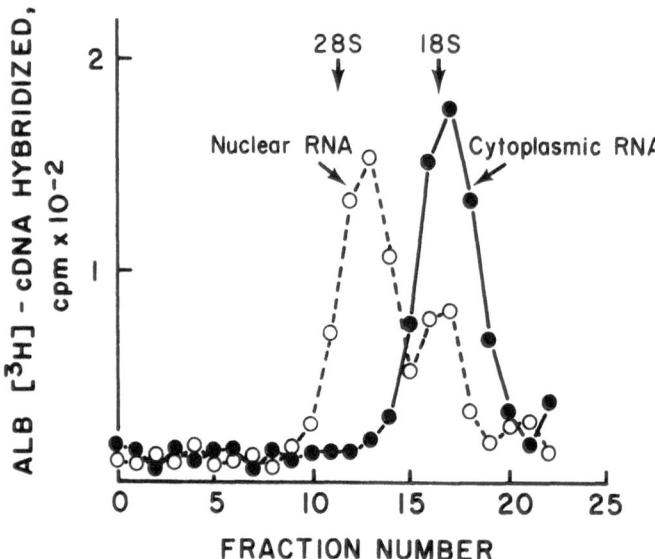

Fig. 13. Identification of higher molecular optional weight nuclear precursor to albumin mRNA by sucrose gradient analysis. In order to identify molecular containing albumin mRNA sequences, hybridization was performed with purified albumin ^{3}H-cDNA and various fractions from an analytical sucrose gradient of liver nuclear RNA under denaturing conditions.

mRNA synthesis, processing, and mRNA release into the cytoplasm, as well as potential abnormalities in these processes. Other possible applications of this technology include cloning of the albumin gene, production of albumin mRNA in bacteria (and perhaps even albumin protein), and a variety of studies on regulation of albumin gene expression. The direct use of this procedure to measure subcellular distribution of albumin mRNA in a variety of pathologic disorders will be presented in Chapter 4.

ACKNOWLEDGMENTS

This research was supported in part by the National Institute of Health Grants AM-17609, AM-17702, AM-16281, Cell and Molecular Biology Training Grant 5-TO1 GM 02209, and Medical Scientist Program Grant 5T32-GM 7288; The Netherlands Organization for Advancement of Pure Research (Z.W.O.) and Niels Stensen Stichting to S.H. Yap; an NIH Research Career Development Award to D.A. Shafritz; and the Irma T. Hisrchl Charitable Trust of New York.

REFERENCES

1. Ancell H: Course of lectures on the physiology and pathology of the blood and the other animal fluids. Lancet 1:222, 1839–1840.
2. Majoor CLH: Over de betekenis van het serum albumine voor de beoordeling en behandeling van inwendige en chirurgische ziekten. Thesis, University of Amsterdam. Scheltema Holkema's Boekhandel en Uitgeversmaatschappij N.V. Amsterdam, 1942.
3. Sterling K: Serum albumin turnover in Laennec cirrhosis as measured by [131] I-albumin. J Clin Invest 30:1228, 1951.
4. Campbell PN, Cuthbertson DP, Mathews CM, McFarlane AS: Behaviours of C- and I-labelled plasma proteins in the rat. Int J Appl Radiol 1:66, 1956.
5. McFarlane AS: Measurements of synthesis rates of liver produced plasma proteins. Biochem J 89:277, 1963.
6. Rothschild MA, Oratz M, Mongelli J, Schreiber SS: Effects of a short term foot on albumin synthesis studies in vivo, in the perfused liver and on amino acid incorporation by hepatic microsomes. J Clin Invest 47:2591, 1968.
7. Shafritz DA: Protein synthesis with messenger ribonucleic acid fractions from membrane-bound and free liver polysomes. J Biol Chem 249:81–88, 1974.
8. Blobel G, Potter VR: Studies on free and membrane-bound ribosomes in rat liver. I. Distribution as related to total cellular RNA, J Mol Biol 26:279–292, 1967.
9. Bloemendal H, Bont MdV, Benedetti EL: Isolation and properties of polyribosomes and fragments of the endoplasmic reticulum from rat liver. Biochem J 103:177–182, 1967.
10. Ramsey, JC Steele WJ: A procedure for the quantitative recovery of homogenous population of undegraded free and membrane-bound polysomes from rat liver. Biochemistry 15:1702–1712, 1976.
11. Yap SH, Strair RK, Shafritz DA: Distribution of rat albumin messenger RNA in membrane-bound versus free polyribosomes as determined by molecular hybridization. Proc Natl Acad USA 74:5397–5401, 1977.
12. Hirsch CA, Hiatt HH: Turnover of liver ribosomes in fed and fasted rats. J Biol Chem 241:5936–5940, 1966.
13. Henshaw EC, Hirsch CA, Morton BE Hiatt: Control of protein synthesis in mammalian tissues through changes in ribosome activity. J Biol Chem 246: 433–446, 1971.
14. Hicks SJ, Drysdale JW, Munro HN: Preferential synthesis of ferritin and albumin by different population of liver polysomes. Science 164:584–585, 1968.
15. Takagi M, Tanaka T, Ogata K: Functional differences in protein synthesis between free and bound polysomes of rat liver. Biochem Biophys Acta 217:148–158, 1970.
16. Shore GC, Tata JR: Two fractions of rough endoplasmic reticulum from rat liver. J Cell Biol 72:726–743, 1977.
17. Redman CM: Biosynthesis of serum proteins and ferritin by free and attached ribosomes of rat liver. J Biol Chem 244:4308–4315, 1969.
18. Shafritz DA, Drysdale JW, Isselbacher KJ: Translation of liver messenger ribonucleic acid in a reticulocyte cell free system. J Biol Chem 248:3220–3227, 1973.
19. Lockard RE, Lingrel JB: The synthesis of mouse hemoglobin chain in rabbit reticulocyte cell free system programmed with mouse reticulocyte 9S RNA. Biochem Biophys Res Commun 37:204–212, 1969.
20. Shafritz DA: Messenger RNA and its translation. In: Protein synthesis, H Weissbach, S Pestka (eds), Acad Press Inc, New York, 556–591, 1977.
21. Mathews MB, Pragnell IM, Osborn M, Arnstein HRV: Stimulation by reticulocyte

initiation factors of protein synthesis in a cell free system from krebs II ascites cells. Biochem Biophy Acta 287:113–123, 1972.

22. Roberts BE, Paterson BM: Efficient translation of tobacco mosaic virus RNA and rabbit 9S globin RNA in a cell free system from commercial wheat germ. Proc Natl Acad Sci USA 70:2330–2334; 1973.

23. Zucker WV, Schulman HM: Stimulation of globin chain initiation by hemin in the reticulocyte cell free system. Proc Natl Acad Sci USA 59:582–589, 1968.

24. Adamson SD, Yau PMP, Herbert E, Zucker WV: Involvement of hemin a stimulatory fraction from ribosomes and a protein synthesis inhibitor in the regulation of hemoglobin synthesis. J Mol Biol 63:247–264, 1972.

25. Gross M, Rabinowitz M: Control of globin synthesis in cell free preparations of reticulocytes by formation of a translational repressor that is inactivated by hemin. Proc Natl Acad Sci USA 69:1565–1568, 1972.

26. Legon S, Jackson RJ, Hunt T: Control of protein synthesis in reticulocyte lysates by hemin. Nature (London) New Biol 241:150–152, 1973.

27. Beuzard Y, London IM: The effects of hemin and double stranded RNA on alpha and beta globin synthesis in reticulocyte and krebs II ascites cell free system and the relationship of these effects to an initiation factor preparation. Proc Natl Acad Sci USA 71:2863–2866, 1974.

28. Atkins JF, Lewis JB, Anderson CW, Gesteland RR: Enhance differential synthesis of proteins in a mammalian cell free system by addition of polyamines. J Biol Chem 250:5688–5695, 1975.

29. Ehrenfeld E, Hunt T: Double-stranded poliovirus RNA inhibit initiation of protein synthesis by reticulocyte lysates. Proc Natl Acad Sci USA 68:1075–1078, 1971.

30. Heywood SM, Kennedy DS, Bester AJ: Separation of specific initiation factors involved in the translation of myosin and myoglobin messenger RNAs and the isolation of new RNA involved in translation Proc Natl Acad Sci USA 741:2428–2431, 1974.

31. Lingrel JB, Lockhard RE, Jones RF, Burr HE, Holder JW: Biologically active messenger RNA for hemoglobin. Ser Haematol 4:37–69, 1971.

32. Neinhuis AW, Canfield PH, Anderson WF: Hemoglobin messenger RNA from human bone marrow. Isolation and translation in homozygous and heterozygous beta-thalasaemia. J Clin Invest 52:1735–1745, 1973.

33. McKeehan WL: Regulation of hemoglobin synthesis. Effect of concentration of messenger ribonucleic acids, ribosome subunits, initiation factors, and salts on ratio of alpha and beta chains synthesized in vitro. J Biol Chem 249:6517–6526, 1974.

34. Palmiter RD: Differential rate of initiation of conalbumin and ovalbumin messenger ribonucleic acid in reticulocyte lysates. J Biol Chem 249:6779–6787, 1974.

35. Sonenshein GE, Brawerman G: Entry of messenger RNA into polyribosomes during recovery from starvation in mouse sarcoma 180 cells. Eur J Biochem 73, 307–312, 1977.

36. Golini F, Thach SS, Birge CH, Safer B, Merrick WC, Thach RE: Competition between cellular and viral mRNA in vitro is regulated by a messenger discriminating initiation factor. Proc Natl Acad Sci USA 73:3040–3044, 1976.

37. Kabat D, Chappell R: Competition between globin messenger ribonucleic acids for a discriminating initiation factor. J Biol Chem 252:2684–2690, 1977.

38. Padilla M, Canaani, D, Groner, Y, Weinstein, JA, Bar-Joseph, M, Merrick, WC, and Shafritz, DA: Initiation Factor eIF-uB (IF-M$_3$) dependent recognition and translation of capped versus uncapped eukaryotic mRNAs. J. Biol Chem in press, 1978.

39. Temin HM, Mizutani S: RNA-dependent DNA polymerase in virions of Rous sarcoma virus. Nature 226:1211–1213, 1970.

40. Baltimore D: RNA-dependent DNA polymerase in virions of RNA tumour viruses. Nature 226: 1209–1211, 1970.

41. Strair RK, YAP SH, Shafritz DA: Use of molecular hybridization to purify and analyze albumin messenger RNA from rat liver. Proc Natl Acad Sci USA 74:4346–4350, 1977.
42. Yap SH, Strair RK, Shafritz DA: Distribution of rat albumin messenger RNA in membrane-bound versus free polyribosomes as determined by molecular hybridization. Proc Natl Acad Sci USA 74:5397–5401, 1977.
43. Bishop JO, Morton JG, Rosbach M, Richardson M: Three abundance classes in HeLa cell messenger RNA. Nature 250:199–204, 1974.
44. Aviv H, Lieder P: Purification of biologically active globin messenger RNA by chromatography on oligothymidylic acid-cellulose. Proc Natl Sci USA 69:1408–1412, 1972.
45. Adesnik M, Salditt M, Thomas W, Darnell JE: Evidence that all messenger RNA molecules (except histone messenger RNA) contain poly (A) sequences and that the poly(A) has a nuclear function. JM. Biol 71:21–30, 1972.
46. Schochetman G, Perry RP: Characterization of messenger RNA released from L cell polyribosomes as a result of temperature shock. J Mol Biol 63:577–590, 1972.
47. Adesnik M, Darnell GE: Biogenesis and characterization of histone messenger RNA in HeLa cells. J Mol Biol 67:397–406, 1972.
48. Rabbitts TH, Milstein C: Mouse immunoglobin genes: studies on the reiteration frequency of light chain genes by hybridization procedures. Eur J Biochem 52:125-133, 1975.
49. Woo SL, Rosen JM, Liarakos CD, Robberson DL, Choi YC, Busch H, Means AR, O'Malley BW: Physical and chemical characterization of purified ovalbumin messenger RNA. J Biol Chem 250:7027–7039, 1975.
50. Suzuki Y, Brown DD: Isolation and identification of the messenger RNA for silk fibroin from Bombyx mori. J Mol Biol 63:409–429, 1972.
51. Venetianer P, Leder P: Enzymatic synthesis of solidphase bound DNA sequences corresponding to specific mammalian genes. Proc Natl Acad Sci USA 71:3892–3895, 1974.
52. Palacios R, Sullivan D, Summers NM, Kiely ML, Schimke RT: Purification of ovalbumin messenger ribonucleic acid by specific immunoadsorption of ovalbumin synthesizing polysomes and millipore partition of ribonucleic acid. J Biol Chem 248:540–548, 1973.
53. Taylor JM, Tse TPH: Isolation of rat albumin messenger RNA. J Biol Chem 251–7461–7467, 1976.
54. Blobel G, Dobberstein B: Transfer of proteins across membranes. I. Presence of proteolytically processed and unprocessed nascent immunoglobulin light chains on membrane-bound ribosomes of murine myeloma. J Cell Biol 67:835–851, 1975.
55. Blobel G, Dobberstein B: Transfer of proteins across membranes. II. Reconstitution of functional rough microsomes from heterologous components. J Cell Biol 67:852–857, 1975.
56. Grubman MJ, Weinstein JA, Shafritz DA: Studies on the mechanism for entry of vesicular stomatitis virus glyco protein G mRNA into membrane-bound polyribosome complexes. J Cell Biol 74:43–57, 1977.
57. Boime I, Boguslowski S, Caine J: The translation of human-placental lactogen mRNA fraction in heterologous cell free system: the synthesis of a possible precursor. Biochem Biophys Res Commun 62:103-109, 1975.
58. Wirth DF, Katz F, Small B, Lodish HF: How a single Sindbis virus mRNA directs the synthesis of one soluble protein and two integral membrane glycoproteins. Cell 10: 253–263, 1977.
59. Katz FN, Rothman JE, Lingappa VR, Blobel G, Lodish HF: Membrane assembly in vitrosynthesis, glycosylation, and asymmetric insertion of a transmembrane protein. Proc Natl Acad Sci USA 74:3278–3282, 1977.

60. Sabatini DD, Tashiro Y, Palade GE: On the attachment of ribosomes to microsomal membranes. J Mol Biol 19:503–524, 1966.
61. Rosbach M, Penman S: Membrane associated protein synthesis of mammalian cells. I. The two classes of membrane associated ribosomes. J Mol Biol 59:227–241, 1971.
62. Tanaka T, Ogata K: Two classes of membrane-bound polyribosomes in rat liver cells and their albumin synthesizing activity. Biochem. Biophys Res Commun 49:1069–1074, 1972.
63. Milcarek C, Penman S: Membrane-bound polyribosomes in HeLa cells: association of polyadenylic acid with membranes. J Mol Biol 89:327–338, 1974.
64. Lande MA, Adesnik M, Sumida M, Tashiro Y, and Sabatini DD: Direct association of messenger RNA with microsomal membranes in human diploid fibroblasts. J Cell Biol 65: 513–528, 1975.
65. Mechler B, Vassalli P: Membrane-bound ribosomes of myeloma cells. III. The role of messenger RNA and the nascent polypeptide chain in the binding of ribosomes to membranes. J Cell Biol 67:25–37, 1975.
66. Judah JD, Nicholls MR: The separation of intracellular serum albumin from rat liver. Biochem J 123:643–648, 1971.
67. Judah JD, Nicholls MR: Biosynthesis of rat serum albumin. Biochem J 123:649–655, 1971.
68. Judah JD, Gamble M, Steadman JH: Biosynthesis of rat serum albumin in rat liver. Evidence for the existance of proalbumin. Biochem J 134:1083–1092, 1973.
69. Russel GH, Geller DM: Rat serum albumin biosynthesis: evidence for a precursor. Biochem Biophys Res Commun 55:239–245, 1973.
70. Russel JH, Geller DM: The structure of rat proalbumin. J Biol Chem 250:3409–3413.
71. Urban J, Inglis AS, Edwards K, Schreiber G: Chemical evidence for the difference between albumin from microsome and serum and a possible precursor product relationship. Biochem Biophys Res Commun 61:494–501, 1974.
72. Edwards K, Schreiber G, Drysburgh H, Urban J, Inglis AS: Synthesis of albumin via precursor protein in cell suspensions from rat liver. Eur J Biochem 63:303–311, 1976.
73. Schreiber G, Urban J, Edwards K, Drysburgh H: Mechanism and regulation of albumin synthesis in liver and hepatomas. Adv Enz Reg 14:163–184, 1974.
74. Schreiber G, Urban G, Edwards K: Possible functions of the oligopeptide extention in the albumin precursor. J Theor Biol 60(01):241–245, 1976.
75. Lundholm K, Lindstedt G, Lunöberg PA, Schersten T: Proalbumin, a precursor in albumin synthesis in human liver tissue. (abstr.) Eur J Clin Invest 6:328, 1976.
76. Strauss AW, Donohue AM, Bennett CD, Rodkey JA, Alberts AW: Rat liver preproalbumin: in vitro synthesis a and partial amino acid sequence. Proc Natl Acad Sci USA 74:1358–1362, 1977.
77. Strair RK, Skoultchi AI, Shafritz DA: A characterization of globin mRNA sequences in the nucleus of duck immature red blood cells. Cell 12:133–141, 1977.

4. Rat liver albumin messenger RNA: subcellular distribution and changes in various models of metabolic diseases

S.H. YAP, R.K. STRAIR, AND D.A. SHAFRITZ

INTRODUCTION

The synthesis of protein requires a complex interaction of cellular constituents. Transfer of genetic information from DNA into protein can be divided into two main processes: 1) transcription of DNA into "messenger" RNA, and 2) translation of "messenger" RNA into specific polypeptide chains composed of the appropriate mixture of amino acids. In differentiated cells this process yields proteins for functions common to all eukaryotic cells ("housekeeping" functions), as well as certain specific proteins with unique properties for the given cell type. For example, the liver is the only organ known to synthesize certain serum proteins, such as albumin, fibrinogen, etc. For the synthesis of these specialized proteins, it is not unreasonable to anticipate that a significant portion of the cellular biosynthetic capacity might be devoted toward synthesis of these specialized proteins. Cellular control processes to regulate synthesis of these proteins at either the transcriptional or post-transciptional level could represent an important mechanism for controlling specialized functions in normal as well as physiologically or pathologically altered cells. In order to assess transcriptional and/or translational events controlling synthesis of unique proteins such as albumin, a simple quantitative assay for messenger RNA was needed.

As mentioned in Chapter 3, previous studies on the detection and quantitation of albumin mRNA have been based primarily on measurements of the ability to synthesize albumin in cell-free systems (1–5). These techniques are at best somewhat indirect and the results may depend on various factors other than the level of a specific mRNA (6, 7, 8). The utilization of radioactively labeled DNA complementary to messenger RNA (under examination) has proved to be most useful for quantitative analysis of a given mRNA and has greatly facilitated studies on regulatory mechanisms in gene expression (9). However, the isolation of the specific mRNA is necessary as a first step in the preparation of a complementary DNA probe.

ISOLATION AND PURIFICATION OF RAT LIVER ALBUMIN mRNA

As mentioned in Chapter 3, a variety of methods have been developed for purification of specific mRNAs from animal cells. Recently, we have developed the technique of immunoprecipitation of albumin synthesizing polysomes in combination with controlled molecular hybridization to prepare highly purified albumin mRNA (10). Details of this purification procedure have been described in Chapter 3. To prove that the purified RNA indeed represents albumin mRNA, we first determined the purity of the RNA by RNA excess hybridization to cDNA transcribed from this RNA. As shown in Fig. 1, the isolated RNA appears as a single frequency component with a $Rot_{1/2}$ of 9.8 $\times$ 10^{-4} mol.-sec/liter (product of RNA

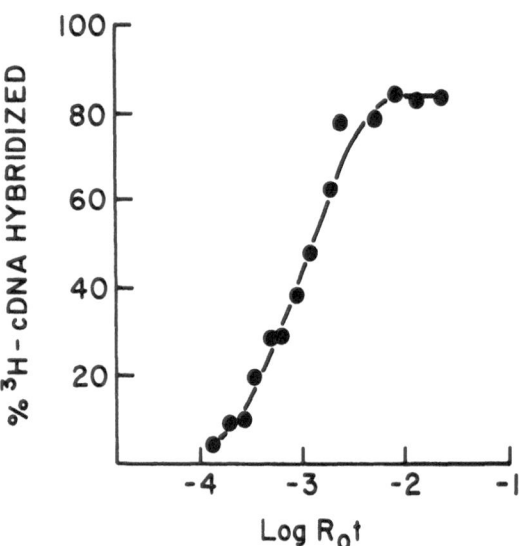

Fig. 1. Hybridization analysis of RNA purified by the technique of immunoprecipitation and controlled molecular hybridization. RNA eluted from immunoprecipitated cDNA-cellulose was hybridized to its homologous cDNA in RNA excess. RNA concentration in these experiments was varied from 0.1 μg/ml to 14 μg/ml. Approximately 2500 cpm of ^{3}H-cDNA was used for each determination.

concentration and incubation time to achieve 50% hybridization of that particular cDNA component). By comparison, the $Rot_{1/2}$ of 6.6×10^{-4} mol.-sec/liter for purified $\alpha + \beta$ globin mRNA, which has a total molecular mass of 4×10^5 daltons, the sequence complexity of the purified RNA is 5.9×10^5 daltons (sum of mass of unique RNA sequences in the RNA preparation). We have also characterized this RNA by sedimentation through a sucrose gradient (Fig. 2). Albumin mRNA either in crude or purified form sediments at 17S and, therefore, has an apparent molecular weight of 6.0×10^5. These results indicate a good agreement between the sequence complexity as determined by molecular hybridization and molecular weight

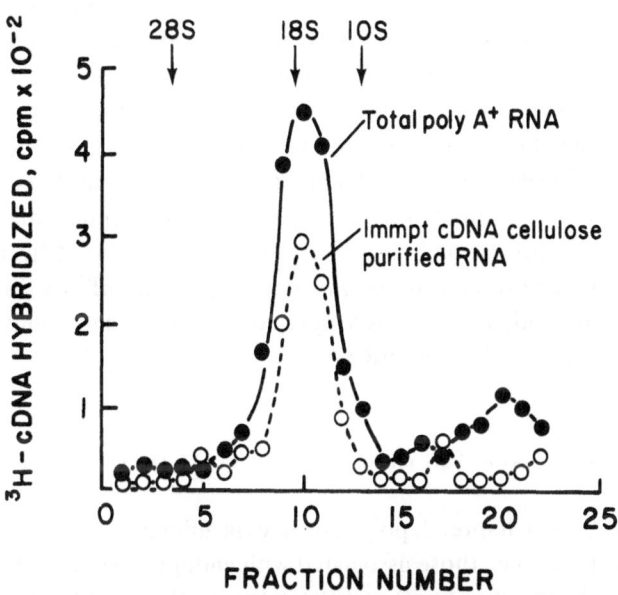

FRACTION NUMBER

Fig. 2. Sucrose gradient analysis of the purified RNA. Cytoplasmic polyadenylated RNA and the purified RNA eluted from the immunoprecipitated cDNA cellulose were sedimented in parallel 5–20% exponential sucrose gradients containing 10 mM Tris-HCl (pH 7.4), 0.5% sodium dodecyl sulfate. Centrifugation was at 23°C for 2 hours at 58,000 rpm in the no. SW61 Ti rotor. Samples were heated to 65°C in 10 mM Tris-HCl (pH 7.4), 0.5% SDS for 5 min. and cooled rapidly on ice prior to application to the gradients. The arrows indicate the position of 28S and 18S ribosomal RNAs and duck reticulocyte 10S globin mRNA in a parallel gradient. Samples from each fraction of the sucrose gradient were either assayed directly or concentrated by ethanol precipitation and assayed for sequences complementary to ³H-cDNA transcribed from the purified RNA. Hybrid formation with fractions of total cytoplasmic poly A⁺ RNA (●—●) or purified RNA (○---○) was detected by incubation with 600 cpm of ³H-cDNA in 5 μl for 40 hours under the conditions as described previously (10).

as determined by sucrose gradient centrifugation. To examine the biological activity of this purified mRNA, we have translated this fraction in a wheat germ cell-free system and have analyzed the cell-free reaction product. The purified RNA actively stimulates incorporation of ^{35}S labeled methionine into hot trichloroacetic acid insoluble polypeptides. Synthesis of "albumin-like" material was demonstrated by indirect immuno-precipitation with rabbit anti-rat serum albumin and goat anti-rabbit gamma globulin. 92% of the ^{35}S methionine labeled polypeptides were precipitated in this system (10). Fig. 3 shows the autoradiogram of a sodium dodecyl sulfate-polyacrylamide slab gel of the cell-free reaction products from the wheat germ system under the direction of purified albumin mRNA (slot e), in comparison to crude total poly A + cytoplasmic RNA (slots b and c) and immunoprecipitated poly A$^+$ RNA (slot d). A comparison of the products synthesized by the various RNAs shows progressive enrichment for a polypeptide which migrates with purified rat serum albumin standard (slot a) (apparent molecular weight $\sim$ 68,000). Under the direction of the purified mRNA (slot e), albumin represents the only detectable high molecular weight component. Furthermore, tryptic peptide analysis (Fig. 4) shows good correlation between standard (in vivo) labeled liver albumin and the cell-free product under direction of purified mRNA. From these studies we concluded that this RNA preparation represents highly purified, biologically active, albumin mRNA.

DISTRIBUTION OF ALBUMIN mRNA IN LIVER CELLS OF FED RATS

As mentioned in Chapter 3, polyribosomes in animal cells can be separated into two populations, those associated with endoplasmic reticulum (membrane-bound polyribosomes) and those free in the cytoplasm (free polyribosomes). Evidence from numerous studies (1,2,4,5,11–16) suggests that secretory proteins are synthesized primarily on membrane-bound polyribosomes, whereas cytosol proteins are synthesized primarily on free polyribosomes. This is not to say that membrane-bound polyribosomes synthesize only secretory proteins or that no membrane proteins are synthesized on free polyribosomes. From these studies, however, it has been concluded that mRNAs for secretory proteins versus cytosol proteins are compartmentalized inside the cell. In the case of albumin, different results have been reported on the intracellular distribution of albumin mRNA (1–5, 14, 15, 16), depending on the system utilized and the methods

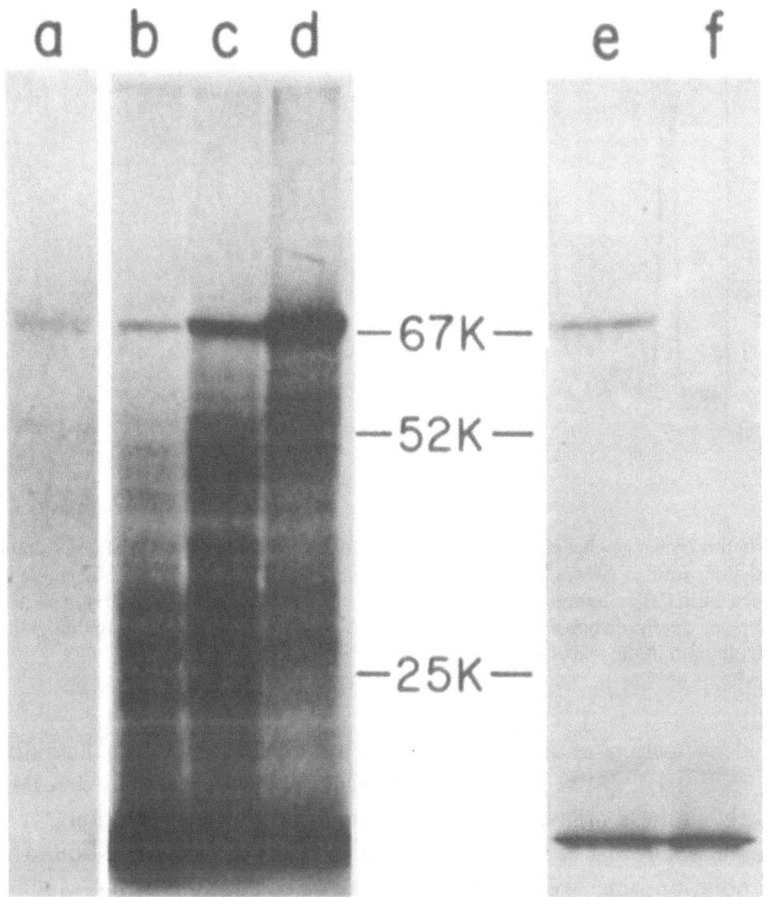

Fig. 3. SDS-polyacrylamide slab gel electrophoresis of cell-free (wheat germ) reaction products. Radioactively labeled in vitro synthesized products under direction of various RNA preparations were analyzed electrophoretically on 10% polyacrylamide-SDS slab gel. Dried slabs were exposed to x-ray film.

slot a, rat serum albumin standard (Coomassie Blue stain)

slot b, cell-free product synthesized under direction of total cytoplasmic poly A⁺ RNA.

slot c, same as b with different preparation of wheat germ extract.

slot d, cell-free product synthesized under direction of poly A⁺ RNA from immuno-precipitated polyribosomes.

slot e, cell-free product synthesized under direction of purified RNA.

slot f, wheat germ extract to which no RNA was added.

The position of VSV protein standards isolated from intact virus (G = 67,000, N = 52,000, M = 25,000) is shown between slots d and e.

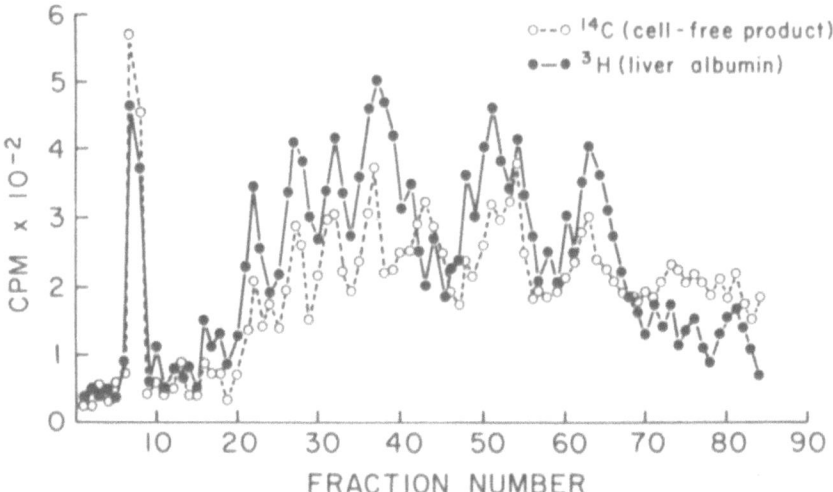

Fig. 4. Ion exchange chromatogram of peptides from the tryptic digestion of (^{14}C) albumin translation product (wheat germ) under direction of purified albumin mRNA and in vivo labelled liver (^{3}H) albumin standard. The close correspondence of each (^{3}H) peak with a (^{14}C) peak clearly demonstrates that the purified albumin mRNA is directing the synthesis of rat albumin in the wheat germ extracts.

for identification and quantitation of the albumin product. Therefore, we have used the technique of molecular hybridization to determine directly albumin mRNA sequence content in subcellular fractions.

As shown in Fig. 5, RNA extracts prepared from membrane-bound and free polyribosomes were utilized for analysis of albumin mRNA sequence content, using albumin ^{3}H-cDNA prepared from purified albumin mRNA (17). In these experiments varying amounts of RNA were titrated against a fix amount of albumin ^{3}H-cDNA. The amount of RNA required to protect for example 50% of albumin ^{3}H-cDNA measures the concentration of albumin mRNA sequence in that fraction. The concentration of albumin mRNA sequences is approximately 16 times greater in membrane-bound polyribosomal RNA than in free polyribosomal RNA. From a standard titration using purified albumin mRNA and labeled albumin cDNA, we compute that 1 pg of purified albumin mRNA protects 5 cpm (counts per minute) of our probe. Therefore, we can determine the absolute amount of albumin mRNA in any RNA fraction by directly measuring cpm of albumin ^{3}H-cDNA protected per unit RNA. In Fig. 5, for example 1 μg of membrane-bound polyribosomal RNA protected 685 cpm of albumin ^{3}H-

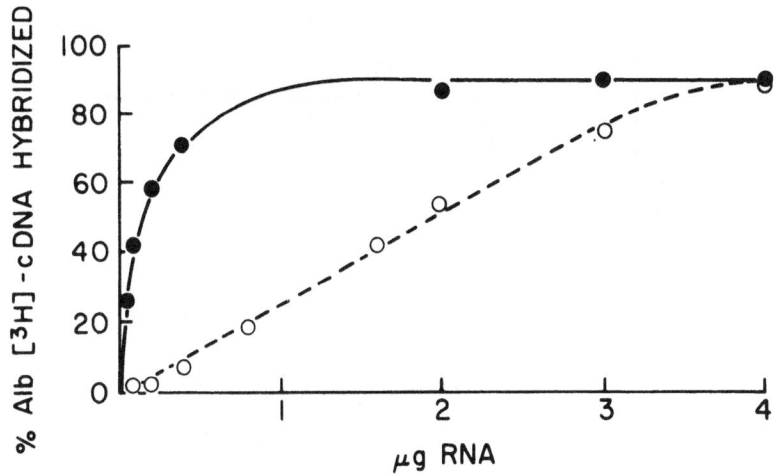

Fig. 5. Hybridization analysis of RNA extracted from membrane-bound and free liver polyribosomes of fed rats. RNA extracted from membranebound (●—●) or free (○---○) polyribosomes was hybridized to a given amount of albumin ^{3}H-cDNA (~400 cpm, spec. activity 7.5 × 10^6 cpm/μg). Reaction conditions were as described previously (10).

cDNA. Therefore, the content of albumin mRNA in this fraction is 137 pg per μg RNA. Free polyribosomal RNA protected 16 times less albumin ^{3}H-cDNA for any given amount of RNA. Therefore, this fraction contains 8.5 pg albumin mRNA per μg RNA.

Since our goal was to quantitate the amount of albumin mRNA in membrane-bound and free polyribosomes, it was particularly important to use isolation procedures which would provide us with high yields of un-degraded polyribosomes. Recently, Ramsey and Steele (18) have developed such a method and we have obtained excellent yields of polyribosomes with this technique (Table 1). Membrane-bound polyribosomes comprise 75–80% of total hepatic polyribosomes. Sucrose gradient analysis established that the polyribosomes were not degraded (Fig. 6). On the basis of this data and our hybridization results (Table 1), it can be calculated that approximately 98% of albumin mRNA in total liver polyribosomes is associated with the membrane-bound fraction. The absolute amount of albumin mRNA in membrane-bound polyribosomes per gram of liver is approximately 564 ng, whereas only 9.5 ng of albumin mRNA per gram of liver is found with free polyribosomes. These results are consistent with the interpretation that mRNA for this secretory protein is segregated in the membrane-bound fraction. However, free cytoplasmic

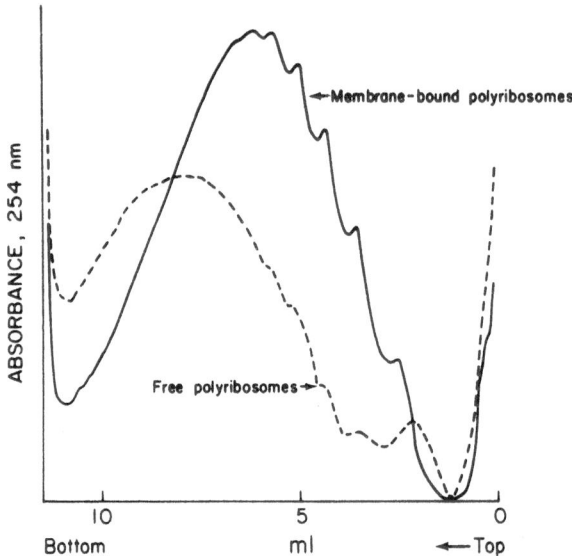

Fig. 6. Sucrose gradient analysis of rat liver membrane-bound and free polyribosomes were layered over 10–40% (w/v) exponential sucrose gradients. After centrifugation at 38,000 rpm in a Beckman no. SW 41 rotor for 65 min. at 2°C, gradients were withdrawn from the bottom of each tube and absorbance at 254 nm monitored with an Altex UV monitor 152.

Table 1. Yield of membrane-bound and free rat liver polyribosomes

Body weight	Liver weight	Polyribosomal membr.-bd.	RNA free	Membrane-bound/ free
(g)	(g)	(mg/g liver)		ratio
205 ± 5	8.5 ± 0.5	3.4	1.2	2.8
300 ± 5	11.5 ± 0.5	5.9	1.2	4.9
215 ± 5	10 ± 2	3.1	1.0	3.1

polyribosomes do contain a low level of albumin mRNA, and it is unclear whether this represents a cross contamination or a fraction of albumin synthesizing polyribosomes in the cytosol prior to their attachment to endoplasmic reticulum membranes.

In numerous studies with mouse and human cells in culture (19–23), it has been observed that most of the mRNA is found in the polyribosome fraction. In normal reticulocytes, however, a significant amount of globin α chain mRNA is present as messenger ribonucleoprotein particles (mRNPs) in the cytosol, whereas globin β chain mRNA is almost exclusively associated with polyribosomes (24, 25). This appears to be related to differential rates of initiation or preferential affinity of β versus α globin mRNAs for the ribosomes. Under special circumstances; e.g. dormant or embryonal cells (26), altered cellular growth conditions (23, 27), or addition of inhibitors of protein synthesis initiation (28), a portion of mRNA may be present in the cytoplasm as mRNPs. Addition of amino acids to starved cells or reversal to normal growth conditions in the presence of an inhibitor of new RNA synthesis (actinomycin D) results in a rapid utilization of mRNPs to form polyribosomes. In liver cells, it has been found that administration of iron in the presence of actinomycin D results in rapid mobilization of ferritin mRNA presumably from messenger RNP in the cytosol (5). Although a direct relationship between supernatant messenger ribonucleoprotein particles and specific protein synthesis has not yet been established, it has been suggested that the occurrence of such extrapolyribosomal mRNA is related to control of protein synthesis. Therefore, information on intracellular distribution of mRNA is important in revealing possible control mechanisms at the level of translation. In this regard we have also determined the portion of total cytoplasmic albumin mRNA present in the postribosomal supernatant fraction. In normal liver only 8.6 ng albumin mRNA per gram of liver (or 1% of total cytoplasmic albumin mRNA) is present in the extrapolyribosomal fraction.

EFFECT OF SHORT TERM FAST ON THE DISTRIBUTION OF ALBUMIN mRNA IN RAT LIVER

In the fasting state, protein synthesis in liver has been found to be reduced both in terms of total activity and activity per unit of polyribosomal RNA (29, 30). These changes are associated with a diminished number of ribosomes and a decrease in the proportion of large polyribosomes. Munro and co-workers have shown that the availability of amino acids is responsible for changes in the hepatic RNA and protein metabolism (31). In rats fed a diet deficient in protein but normal in caloric intake, there is a marked decrease in RNA and protein levels in the liver (32). The amount of intracellular albumin is also reduced in fasted rats (Table 2). Based on in vivo and in vitro studies, it has been reported that albumin synthesis also decreases very rapidly during starvation (33, 34). These decreased rates of albumin and protein synthesis are associated with disaggregation primarily

Table 2. Intracellular albumin level in fed vs. fasted rat liver

Cell fraction		Albumin/liver (µg/g)
Cytosol	Fed	103
	Fasted	109
Microsomal	Fed	273
	Fasted	211

of membrane-bound polyribosomes. There is also an increase in RNA breakdowns (29, 35). In our studies (36), we have demonstrated that the disaggregation of membrane-bound polysomes during starvation is accompanied by a decreased concentration of albumin mRNA content per unit of polyribosomal RNA. As shown in Table 3, the amount of poly-ribosomal albumin mRNA is increased 18 fold. Further studies indicate that the extrapolyribosomal albumin mRNA sequences are present in the cytosol as intact albumin mRNA molecules (sedimenting at 17S, Fig. 7). These complexes sediment as a braod peak and are predominantly con-tained between 30S and 50S (Fig. 8), which suggests that albumin mRNA molecules released from polyribosomes during starvation may be present in the cytoplasm as messenger RNP.

Previously, Kirsh et al. (33), Sidransky et al. (37), and Rothschild et al. (34) showed that the reduced rate of albumin synthesis in starvation can be reversed very rapidly by supplementation with food or amino

Table 3. Distribution of albumin mRNA sequences in liver subcellular fractions from fed vs. starved rats

		Polyribosomes membrane-bound	Free	Postribosmal super.
Alb. mRNA seq. (% total alb. mRNA)	Fed	97	2	1
	Starved	31.4	8.6	60
Alb. mRNA content (ng/g liver)	Fed	582	6.9	8.6
	Starved	132	9.4	220
Alb. mRNA conc. (pg/µg RNA)	Fed	130	7	13
	Starved	37	11	600

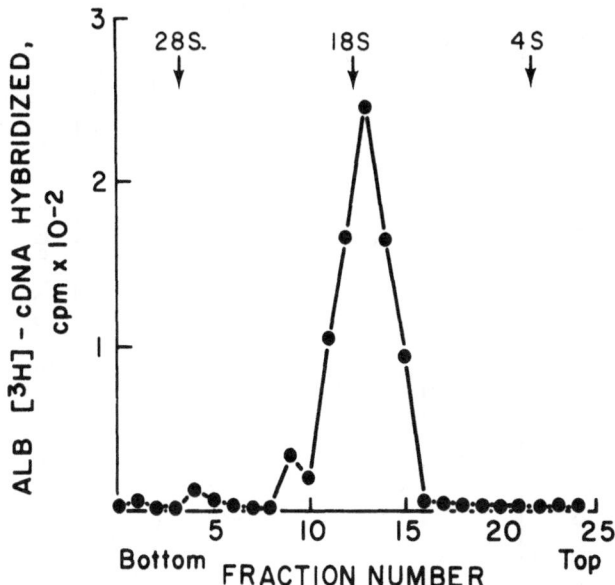

Fig. 7. Sucrose gradient analysis of the liver RNA prepared from the postribosomal supernatant fraction of starved rats. After treatment of the postribosomal supernatant (obtained from the experiment described in Fig. 8) with proteinase K (1 mg/ml) in 0.1M NaCl, 0.5% SDS, 10 mM Tris-HCl pH 7.6, 1 mM EDTA, the RNA was sedimented in an 15-30% exponential sucrose gradient containing 10 mM Tris-HCl pH 7.4, 0.5% SDS. Centrifugation was at 38,000 rpm for 2 hours at 23°C. The arrows indicate the position of 28S and 18S ribosomal RNAs and duck reticulocyte 10S globin mRNA in a parallel gradient. Other experimental procedures are the same as described in Figure 2.

acids. At the same time there is rapid assembly of polyribosomes. Therefore, it seems that reactivation of albumin mRNA occurs during recovery. Although there is no direct evidence at present to prove that the cytosol albumin mRNA is taken up into polyribosomes during recovery, as has been shown in mouse and human cultured cells (23, 27, 28), the above experiments are consistent with such an hypothesis.

INFLUENCE OF CHRONIC RENAL FAILURE ON THE DISTRIBUTION OF ALBUMIN mRNA IN RAT LIVER

Previously, we have shown that in rats with chronic renal failure (blood urea nitrogen greater than 45 mg/100 ml, normal <25, and serum creatinine higher than 1.2 mg/100 ml, normal <0.5, one month after surgical

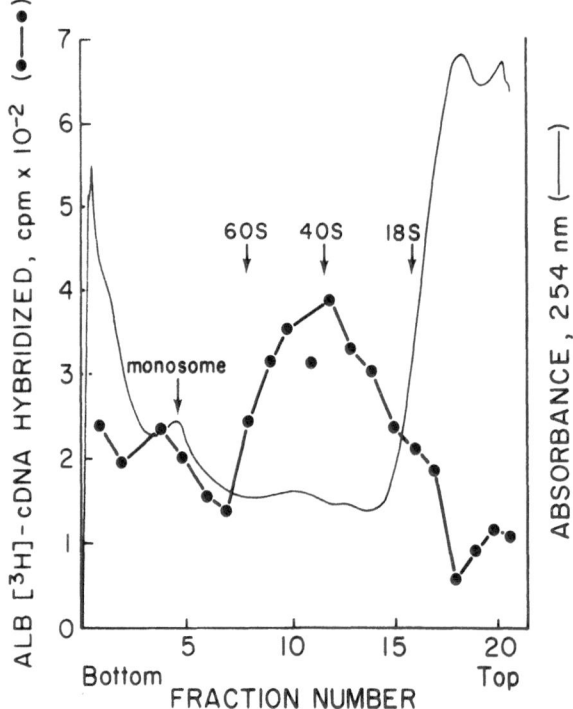

Fig. 8. Sucrose gradient analysis of the postribosomal supernatant fraction prepared from liver of starved rats. 400 μl of 131,000Xg (12 min.) supernatant fraction (equivalent to 3.3 A_{260} units (RNA) prepared from liver of starved rats as previously described (36), was layered over a 12 ml, 10–40% (w/v) exponential sucrose gradient. Centrifugation was performed in a Beckman no. SW 41 rotor at 38,000 rpm for 2 hrs. at 2°C. Gradients were withdrawn from the bottom of each tube and absorbance monitored at 254 nm. RNA from each fraction was then prepared by proteinase K digestion as described in Fig. 6 and ethanol precipitated. After centrifugation RNA pellet from each fraction was re-suspended in 50 μl de-ionized distilled water and each fraction analyzed for albumin mRNA sequence content as described in Fig. 2.

reduction in renal mass), cell-free protein synthesis is reduced 30–40% in liver membrane-bound polyribosomes (38). Protein synthesis activity of free polyribosomes remains normal (Table 4). Albumin synthesis by membrane-bound polyribosomes in uremia is decreased even more than the reduction in total protein synthesis (50% reduction). These changes are associated with a decrease in average size primarily of membrane-bound polyribosomes in uremic animals and an increase in the intracellular level of albumin. We also reported that the increased concentration of

Table 4. Synthesis of "Albumin-like" material by liver membrane-bound and free polysomes from control vs. uremic rats

Polyribosomes		Protein synthesis (cpm/μg RNA)	"Albumin" synthesis (cpm/μg RNA)
Membrane-bound	Control	3570	135
	Uremic	2800	58
Free	Control	6140	51
	Uremic	8220	46

intracellular albumin was found in the cytosol fraction. However, more recently, using more gentle technique of liver perfusion and cellular homogenization, we find that this extra albumin is present in the microsomal fraction. Therefore, it appears that membrane vescicles containing albumin from liver of uremic animals are more fragile than normal liver vescicles. We have no idea whether this is related to the abnormalities in protein synthesis in the membrane-bound polyribosome fraction.

Although there is disaggregation primarily of membrane-bound polyribosomes in liver of uremic rats, the albumin mRNA concentration is not decreased (Table 5). In actual fact the albumin mRNA content in the membrane-bound fraction of uremic rats is increased by 59% per gram of liver compared to control animals (Table 5). The content of albumin

Table 5. Distribution of albumin mRNA sequences in liver polyribosomes from control vs. uremic rats

		Polyribosome fraction	
		Membrane-bound	Free
Alb.mRNA seq. (% total alb. mRNA)	Control	97	3
	Uremia	98	2
Alb.mRNA content (ng/g liver)	Control	548	16
	Uremia	873	20
Conc. alb. mRNA (pg/μg liver)	Control	146	18
	Uremia	146	18

mRNA in free polyribosomes is essentially unchanged. This accumulation of albumin mRNA in the membrane-bound polyribosome fraction, associated with a generalized decrease in albumin synthesis, suggests that there is a block in protein synthesis at the level of translation. These findings are in contrast to results obtained with fasted rats (Table 3), and indicated a separate mechanism for the abnormality in albumin metabolism in these two conditions. Although the exact mechanism for the translational block in uremia is not clear, the finding of increase intravesicular albumin might reflect a dysfunction of albumin secretion.

DISTRIBUTION OF ALBUMIN mRNA IN LIVER CIRRHOSIS INDUCED WITH CARBON-TETRACHLORIDE

Hypoalbuminaemia commonly occurs in patients with liver cirrhosis (39, 40, 41), a disease which is characterized by distorted hepatic architecture. For many years the hypoalbuminaemia had been ascribed to an impairment of the albumin synthesizing capability of the damaged liver (42, 43). However, in recent years it has become clear that a normal or increased albumin synthesis can also be found in patients with liver cirrhosis and hypoalbuminaemia (41, 44). In the experimental studies of liver cirrhosis induced in young rats by repeated intraperitoneal injections of carbon-tetrachloride, it was observed that the capability of the liver to synthesize albumin in vivo and in vitro is not impaired (45, 46). We, therefore, designed studies to investigate whether there was a compensatory increase in the level of albumin mRNA to account for normal albumin synthesis in cirrhotic liver.

Male Spraque-Dawley rats initially weighing 50 to 100 g were divided into two groups. The first served as control and the second group was injected intraperitoneally with 0.15 ml carbon tetrachloride in mineral oil (1:7, v/v) 3 times per week. This procedure generally induced liver cirrhosis after 7 weeks. All animals were fed ad libitum with commercial purina chow food pellets. One week after the last injection of CCl_4, control and experimental animals were sacrificed and the livers removed and processed for isolation of polyribosomes as previously described (17). The livers of CCl_4 treated animals were firm and invariably enlarged (average liver weight 18 grams in experimental animals versus 15 g in controls). The histopathological findings correspond to a moderate stage of cirrhosis with an intense inflammatory cell infiltration. As shown in Table 6, the

Table 6. Distribution of albumin mRNA sequences in liver polyribosomal fractions from control vs. cirrhotic rats

| | | *Polyribosomal fraction* | |
		Membrane-bound	*Free*
Alb. mRNA seq. (% total alb. mRNA)	Control	98	2
	Cirrhotic	97	3
Alb. mRNA content (ng/g liver)	Control	316	5
	Cirrhotic	298	8
Alb. mRNA conc. (pg/μg RNA)	Control	122	8
	Cirrhotic	122	16

concentration of albumin mRNA in free as well as in membrane-bound polyribosomal RNA of cirrhotic liver was unchanged compared to control animals. The content of albumin mRNA per gram of liver is slightly lower in cirrhosis, but the total content of albumin mRNA per liver is essentially the same in the two groups. From this study we can conclude that although cell damages exist in experimental cirrhosis, the content of albumin mRNA in the liver is normal.

SUMMARY

Based on the experimental approach of immunoprecipitation of specific polyribosomes containing nascent chains for albumin and controlled molecular hybridization, we have been able to purify biological active albumin mRNA from rat liver. Using labeled albumin cDNA, transcribed in reverse from purified albumin mRNA, we have determined the content and distribution of albumin mRNA in subcellular fractions of rat liver in various models of metabolic diseases. This technique in conjunction with measurements of cell-free protein synthesis and intracellular albumin levels has allowed us to make considerable progress in understanding the molecular pathophysiology of albumin metabolism in the liver. With these techniques we should also be able to determine the molecular basis for the changes of hepatic albumin synthesis in other experimental models, and this same approach should enable us to study a wide variety of control processes operating to regulate expression of the albumin gene.

ACKNOWLEDGEMENTS

This research was supported in part by National Institute of Health Grants AM-17609, AM-17702 and AM-16281, Cell and Molecular Biology Training Grant 5-TO1 GM-02209 and Medical Scientist Program Grant 5T32 GM-7288; the Netherlands Organization for Advancement of Pure Research (Z.W.O.) and Niels Stensen Stichting to S.H. Yap, an NIH Research Career Development Award to D.A. Shafritz; and the Irma T. Hirschl Charitable Trust of New York.

REFERENCES

1. Takagi M, Tanaka T, Ogata K: Functional differences in protein synthesis between free and bound polysomes of rat liver. Biochem Biophys Acta 217:148–158, 1970.
2. Hicks SJ, Drysdale JW, Munro HN: Preferential synthesis of ferritin and albumin by different population of liver polysomes. Science 164:584–585, 1960.
3. Shafritz DA: Evidence for nontranslated messenger ribonucleic acid in membrane-bound and free polysomes in rabbit liver. J Biol Chem 249:89–93, 1974.
4. Shore GC, Tata JR: Two fractions of rough endoplasmic reticulum from rat liver. J Cell Biol 72:726–743, 1977.
5. Zähringer J, Baliga BS, Drake RL, Munro HN: Distribution of ferritin mRNA and albumin mRNA between free and membrane-bound rat liver polysomes. Biochem Biophys Acta 474:234–244, 1977.
6. Shafritz DA: Messenger RNA and its translation. In: Protein synthesis, H Weissbach, S Pestka (eds), Molecular Biology Series, B Horecker (ed), Acad Press, New York, 555–601, 1977.
7. Peterson JA: An assay for albumin messenger RNA in a vitro protein synthesizing system from wheat germ. Nucleic Acids Res 3: 1427–1436, 1976.
8. Tse TPH, Taylor JM: Translation of albumin messenger RNA in a cell free protein synthesizing system derived from wheat germ. J Biol Chem 252:1272–1278, 1977.
9. Harris SE, Rosen JM, Means AR, O'Malley BW: Use of a specific probe for ovalbumin messenger RNA to quantitate estrogen-induced gene transcripts. Biochemistry 14:2072–2081, 1975.
10. Strair RK, Yap SH, Shafritz DA: Use of molecular hybridization to purify and analyze albumin messenger RNA from rat liver. Proc Natl Acad Sci USA 74:4346–4350, 1977.
11. Siekevitz P, Palade G: A cytochemical study of the pancreas of the guinea pig V. In vivo incorporation of leucine -L- C¹⁴ into the chymotrypsinogen of various cell fractions. J Biophys Biochem Cytol 7:619–630, 1960.
12. Birbeck MSC, Mercer EH: Cytology of cells which synthesize protein. Nature 189:558–560, 1961.
13. Peters T Jr: The biosynthesis of rat serum albumin. Properties of rat albumin and its occurrence in liver cell fractions. J Biol Chem 237:1181–1185, 1962.
14. Redman CM: Biosynthesis of serum proteins and ferritin by free and attached ribosomes of rat liver. J Biol Chem 244:4308–4315, 1969.
15. Uenoyama K, Ono T: Specificities in messenger RNA and ribosomes from free and bound polyribosomes. Biochem Biophys Res Comm 49:713–719, 1972.
16. Rolleston FS: Membrane-bound and free ribosomes. Sub-cell Biochem 3:91–117, 1974.
17. Yap SH, Strair RK, Shafritz DA: Distribution of rat albumin messenger RNA in membrane-bound versus free polyribosomes as determined by molecular hybridization. Proc Natl Acad Sci USA 74, 1977.
18. Ramsey JC, Steele WJ: A procedure for the quantitative recovery of homogeneous

population of undegraded free and membrane-bound polysomes from rat liver. Biochemistry 15:1704–1712, 1976.

19. Lee SY, Krsmanovic V, Braverman G: Initiation of polysome formation in mouse sarcoma 180 ascites cells. Utilization of cytoplasmic messenger ribonucleic acid. Biochemistry 10:895–900, 1971.

20. Vaughan MH, Pawlowski PJ, Forchhammer T: Regulation of protein synthesis initiation in HeLa cells deprived of single essential amino acids. Proc Natl Acad Sci USA 68:2057–2061, 1971.

21. Van Venroy WJW, Henshaw EC, Hirsch CA: Effects of deprival of glucose or individual amino acids on polyribosome distribution and rate of protein synthesis in cultured mammalian cells. Biochem Biophs Acta 259:127–137, 1972.

22. Hogan BLM, Konner A: Ribosomal subunits of Landschütz ascites cells during changes in polysome distribution. Biochem Biophys Acta 169:129–138, 1968.

23. Sonenshein GE, Braverman G: Entry of mRNA into polyribosomes during recovery from starvation in mouse sarcoma 180 cells. Eur J Biochem 73:307–312, 1977.

24. Olsen GD, Gaskill P, Kabat D: Presence of hemoglobin messenger ribonucleoprotein in a reticulocyte supernatant fraction. Biochem Biophys Acta 272:299–304, 1972.

25. Jacobs-Lorena M, Baglioni C: Messenger RNA for globin in the postribosomal supernatant of rabbit reticulocytes. Proc Natl Acad Sci USA 69:1425–1428, 1972.

26. Dworkin MB, Rudensey LM, Infante AA: Cytoplasmic nonpolysomal ribonucleoprotein particles in sea urchin embryos and their relationship to protein synthesis. Proc Natl Acad Sci USA 74:2223–2235, 1977.

27. Schochetman G, Perry RP: Characterization of the messenger RNA released from L cell polyribosomes as a result of temperature shock. J Mol Biol 63:577–590, 1972.

28. Vesco C, Colombo B: Effect of sodium fluoride on protein synthesis in HeLa cells: inhibitions of ribosome dissociation. J Mol Biol 49:335–352 1970.

29. Hirsch CA, Hiatt HH: Turnover of liver ribosomes in fed and fasted rats. J Biol Chem 241:5936–5940, 1966.

30. Henshaw EC, Hirsch CA, Morton BE, Hiatt HH: Control of protein synthesis in mammalian tissues through changes in ribosome activity. J Biol Chem 246:436–446, 1971.

31. Munro HN, Naismith DJ, Wikramanayake TW: The influence of energy intake on ribonucleic acid metabolism. Biochem J 54:198–205, 1953.

32. LePage GA, Potter VR, Busch H, Heidelberger C, Hurlbert RB: Growth of Carcinoma implants in fed and fasted rats. Cancer Res 12, 153–157, 1952.

33. Kirsch R, Frith L, Black E, Hoffenberg R: Regulation of albumin synthesis and catabolism by alteration of dietary protein. Nature 217: 578–579, 1968.

34. Rothschild MA, Oratz M, Mongelli J, Schreiber SS: Effect of short-term fast on albumin synthesis studied in vivo, in the perfused liver and on amino acid incorporation by hepatic microsomes. J Clin Invest 47:2591–2599 (1968).

35. Staehelin T, Verney E, Sidransky H: The influence of nutritional change on polyribosomes of the liver. Biochem Biophys Acta 145:105–119, 1967.

36. Yap SH, Strair RK, Shafritz DA: Effect of a short-term fast on the distribution of cytoplasmic albumin messenger RNA in rat liver. J Biol Chem 1978.

37. Sidransky H, Sarma DSR, Bongiorno M, Verney E: Effect of dietary tryptophan on hepatic polyribosomes and protein synthesis in fasted mice. J Biol Chem 243:1123–1132, 1968.

38. Grossman SB, Yap SH, Shafritz DA: Influence of chronic renal failure on protein synthesis and albumin metabolism in rat liver. J Clin Invest 59:869–878, 1977.

39. Gutman AB: The plasma proteins in disease. Advances in Protein Chemistry 4:155–250, 1948.

40. Hash E, Jarnum S, Tygstrup N: Albumin synthesis rate as a measure of liver function in

patients with cirrhosis. Acta Med Scand 182:83–92, 1967.
41. Rothschild MA, Oratz M, Zimmon D, Schreiber SS, Weiner I, Caneghem AV: Albumin synthesis in cirrhotic subjects with ascites studied with carbonate ^{14}C. J Clin Invest 48:344–350, 1969.
42. Post J, Patek AJ: Serum proteins in cirrhosis of the liver. Arch Intern Med 69:67–82, 83–89, 1942.
43. Jones EA: Symposium on physiology and pathophysiology of plasma protein metabolism. Hans Huber Publications, Berne, 12-61, 1969.
44. Yap SH: The rates of synthesis and degradation of albumin in man in normal and pathological circumstances, Thesis, University of Nijmegen, The Netherlands, 1976.
45. Chandrasekharan N: A study of albumin synthesis and some biochemical changes in nutritional cirrhosis of the liver. Aust J exp Biol Med Sci 49:383–395, 1971.
46. Rojkind M, Kershenobich D: Effect of colchicine on collagen, albumin and transferrin synthesis by cirrhotic rat liver slices. Biochem Biophys Acta 378:415–423, 1975.

5. Regulation of albumin synthesis

M. Oratz, M.A. Rothschild, and
S.S. Schreiber

During the past few years, much has been learned about the basic bio-synthesis of serum albumin. This protein, which now occupies so much of the liver's productive capacity in terms of an exported protein, exists intracellularly in two forms, pro-albumin and albumin. The latter is identical to serum albumin, while the former is an albumin molecule containing either a pentapeptide or hexapeptide attached to the amino terminus of albumin (1, 2). This small peptide moiety is removed by an intracellular protease at some time following synthesis and just prior to secretion (3). More recently, it has been demonstrated that the initial albumin molecule synthesized contains eighteen additional amino acids attached to the small peptide moiety of proalbumin (4). It may well be that this peptide extension on proalbumin is the signal peptide necessary for the interaction of the large ribosomal subunit with the endoplasmic reticulum allowing for transfer of the nascent albumin chain across the endoplasmic membrane with subsequent proteolysis of the signal peptide to form the proalbumin (5). It is of interest that the amino acid sequence in the peptide extension of the pre and pro albumin molecule is quite equivalent to sequences in other precursor molecules for proteins whose eventual destiny is export from some other cellular organ (6).

The biosynthesis of albumin may operationally be divided into 3 regulatable areas:

1. RNA
2. Translation
3. Intracellular processing

Area no. 1, RNA: Before albumin can be synthesized, the necessary machinery for its synthesis has to be assembled. The synthesizing organelle, the polysome, is composed of ribosomes (r-RNA), the messenger RNA (m-RNA) for albumin, and the 20 transfer RNAs (t-RNA) for the individual amino acids present in albumin. Within the hepatocyte there are many m-RNAs for other proteins competing for the limited amount of ribosomes present so that any factor that affects RNA synthesis must have an effect on albumin synthesis.

Area no. 2, Translation: The assembly of the precursor albumin molecule occurs in this area. Since albumin is a secreted protein a signal peptide has to be synthesized in order to form an endoplasmic reticulum bound polysome, thereafter, the rest of the protein molecule is synthesized. This area is very sensitive to amino acid availability, particularly arginine which is normally present in trace quantities in the liver. Area no. 3, Intracellular processing: The growing peptide chain is inserted through the large ribosomal subunit into the endoplasmic reticulum cisternae and transported to the Golgi apparatus and then transported into the bloodstream by ill-defined mechanisms. During its passage to the Golgi, proteolytic cleavage occurs converting the pre-proalbumin into proalbumin and albumin. Thus, the comments that shall review the basic data concerning the influences of various stresses (Table 1) on the rates of albumin synthesis must be interpreted in the light of these observations.

It is not known whether nutrition, hormones, or toxic stresses interfere with the pre and proalbumin sequences made on the free polysome population or whether they influence the rates of synthesis after the albumin molecule has started on its synthetic pathway on the endoplasmic membrane bound polysome. It is hoped that comments in other sections of this text will throw light on this most fascinating observation.

NUTRITION

Perhaps the most important factor influencing the rate of albumin synthesis is nutrition (7–12). It has been clearly shown that as much as a 24 hr fast will

Table 1. Factors which influence albumin synthesis

1. Nutrition
2. Hormones
3. Ethanol and other hepatotoxins
4. Disease
5. Colloid osmotic pressure
6. Environment

rapidly reduce the total hepatic cellular RNA by means of increasing the rate of degradation of RNA and decreasing its synthesis (11). After a short period of time, these two processes again come into balance. However, the hepatic cellular RNA may well be reduced at this point by one-third. Most of this reduction is, obviously, ribosomal RNA, the major fraction of cellular RNA (13). Associated with fasting is a significant decrease in the degree of aggregation of the endoplasmic membrane bound polysome: that is, the number of ribosomal subunits capable of translating the message are decreased in number and therefore the organelle is not an efficient synthesizing mechanism (14).

The cause of the disaggregation of the bound polysome is two fold. Fasting decreases r-RNA and consequently the number of ribosomes available for combination with m-RNA. Further, upon completion of a peptide chain the ribosome disengages from the m-RNA and if an adequate supply of the rate limiting amino acid is not present, protein synthesis cannot continue and translocation of the ribosome on the m-RNA is halted. This would prevent additional ribosomes from combining with m-RNA giving rise to a disaggregated polysome.

Just as a fast inhibits the rate of production of albumin, so does refeeding rapidly restore albumin production to normal levels. In isolated perfused liver studies, it has been demonstrated that specific amino acids added in excess to the perfusate of livers from fasted donors can result in stimulation of albumin synthesis and in reaggregation of the endoplasmic membrane bound polysome (14) (Table 2).

In many instances the level of albumin production was higher than that seen in livers from fed animals. This result could be due to the stability and long life of the m-RNA for albumin production and thus there is less competition with other short lived m-RNAs for the limited number of ribosomes. These amino acids, including ornithine which is not incorporated into albumin, that stimulate albumin synthesis, also stimulate urea production. An increased urea production requires that an increased quantity of arginine be generated and also results in an increased production of ornithine. Ornithine is not only an important intermediate in the urea cycle but also is the immediate precursor of putrescine which in turn is the immediate precursor of the polyamines spermidine and spermine (Fig. 1.) These polyamines have been shown to play important roles in the maintenance of the integrity of the polysomal system (15, 16) and, more recently, it has been shown that the stimulation of polyphenylalanine synthesis by spermidine is due mainly to the stimulation of initiation of polypeptide

Table 2. Effect of amino acids on albumin synthesis

Donor	Perfusate	Urea synthesis mg/100 g/hr.	Albumin synthesis mg/100 g/hr.
Fed	Control	34 ± 6^a	16 ± 1
Fasted	Control	42 ± 4	8 ± 1
	Trp	55 ± 3	18 ± 4
	Arg	122 ± 10	19 ± 2
	Orn	60 ± 6	17 ± 2
	Phe	93 ± 7	20 ± 3
	Lys	63 ± 5	20 ± 2
	Gln	230 ± 42	12 ± 1
	Thr	48 ± 5	13
	Ala	67 ± 3	15 ± 1
	Pro	60 ± 6	18 ± 3
	Leu	19 ± 5	5 ± 2
	Val	34 ± 5	9 ± 1
	Met	29 ± 4	7 ± 1
	His	25 ± 3	8 ± 1

[a] All values are expressed as mean ± SEM.

PATHWAYS OF ORNITHINE METABOLISM

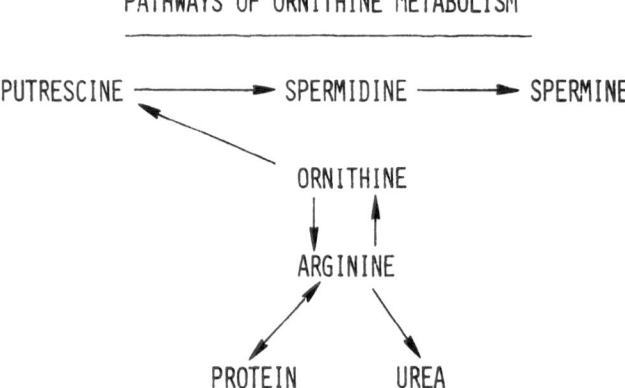

Fig. 1. Schematic representation of two pathways of ornithine metabolism.

synthesis (17). Not all amino acids are effective in stimulating albumin and urea synthesis in the isolated perfused liver system, for leucine, valine, methionine and histidine fail to result in the stimulation of either urea or albumin synthesis (14) (Table 2). Thus, it appears that the urea cycle and albumin synthesis are more intimately connected than was heretofore imagined.

HORMONAL

The actions of the various hormones are clearly interrelated and probably have as an underlying basic mechanism the stimulation of RNA synthesis. Certainly excess thyroid and cortisone, both experimentally and under clinical conditions, have been shown to result in marked increments in the rates of albumin synthesis, as well as in the rates of albumin degradation, without significant alteration in the total exchangeable albumin pool (18, 19). These two hormones also result in significant changes in RNA metabolism with a lack of thyroid hormone resulting in a lowered messenger and ribosomal RNA synthesis, and cortisone stimulating the synthesis of nuclear, transfer and ribosomal RNA. Nitrogen accumulates within the liver as long as the diet is adequate, and cortisone may in fact promote binding of the ribosomes to the endoplasmic reticulum (20–29).

Growth hormone is another hormone whose effects on protein synthesis is mediated via RNA synthesis. Growth hormone has been shown to increase r-RNA synthesis (30) as well as m-RNA synthesis (31, 32). Hypophysectomy has been shown to result in a 50% decrease in albumin m-RNA activity in rates (33), whereas growth hormone replacement in hypophysectomized rats restored albumin synthesis (34, 35).

The lack of insulin in experimental animals results in a loss of the endoplasmic reticulum, while protein synthesis has been shown to be stimulated by insulin (36, 37). However, diabetes as a disease is not necessarily associated with an altered rate of albumin synthesis. How the hormones act and where they act in the albumin synthetic scheme is clearly not known. Probably a fine balance between the various hormones and the nutritional state of the animal is required for the optimal setting for all protein synthesis.

ETHANOL AND OTHER TOXINS

The acute and chronic effects of ethanol exposure on the hepatic protein synthesizing systems are receiving more and more attention. Acute exposure to ethanol has been shown to clearly result in a disruption of the endoplasmic membrane (38). There is a rapid loss in the ability to synthesize serum albumin, and the combination of altered nutrition and ethanol exposure in the isolated perfused liver systems is more toxic to the albumin synthesizing mechanism than either stress alone (14). There is a minimal retention of albumin or precursor within the liver cell, but this amounts to only a miniscule fraction of the normal albumin synthetic rate. Excess amino acids, spermine, and in particular arginine plus spermine, has been shown to be able to reduce and ameliorate the acute effects of ethanol on the albumin synthesizing system in isolated perfused liver studies (39) (Table 3). It has been suggested that acetaldehyde, the primary product of ethanol metabolism, is the toxic agent responsible for the effects of ethanol. While acetaldehyde is toxic to the albumin synthetic mechanism in livers from fed donors, it is not toxic in livers from fasted donors, and with the use of 4-methyl pyrazole, an agent which inhibits ethanol oxidation to acetaldehyde, it has been shown that acetaldehyde cannot explain the inhibitory effects of ethanol on albumin synthesis (Table 4). Moreover, the mode of action of ethanol and acetaldehyde is different. In the presence of ethanol, albumin synthesis is inhibited coincident with disaggregation of the bound polysome, while acetaldehyde is effective without disaggregating the bound polysome. It is more likely that there is some intermediate metabolic step in the total metabolic degradation of ethanol through acetaldehyde to acetate, which is responsible not only for the altered rates of albumin and urea synthesis seen following ethanol exposure, but also for the disruption of the endoplasmic reticulum.

Table 3. Alcohol and albumin synthesis in perfused rabbit liver

Donor	Perfusate	Urea synthesis mg/100 g/hr.	Albumin synthesis mg/100 g/hr.	% Polysome aggregation [a]
Fed	Control	32 ± 3 [e]	17 ± 2	69
	Alc [b]	11 ± 2	6 ± 1	28
	Alc + Spe [c]	20 ± 2	9 ± 1	46
	Alc + Arg [d]	28 ± 4	12 ± 1	53
Fasted	Control	62 ± 6	9 ± 1	48
	Spe	74 ± 7	10 ± 1	65
	Arg + Spe	208 ± 38	16 ± 3	60
	Alc	20 ± 4	5 ± 1	5
	Alc + Spe	29 ± 4	9 ± 1	43
	Alc + Arg	34 ± 7	6 ± 1	5
	Alc + Arg + Spe	87 ± 14	13 ± 2	48

[a] Polysomes containing more than 3 ribosomes.
[b] Alc = ethanol 200 mg ".
[c] Spe = spermine 1 mM
[d] Arg = Arginine 10 mM
[e] All values are expressed as mean $\pm$ SEM.

Table 4. Comparison of the effects of alcohol and acetaldehyde on albumin synthesis in perfused rabbit liver

Donor	Perfusate	Urea synthesis mg/100 g/hr.	Albumin synthesis mg/100 g/hr.	% Polysome[a] aggregation
Fed	Control	32 ± 3[e]	17 ± 2	69
	Alc[b]	11 ± 2	6 ± 1	28
	Alc + 4-MP[c]	20 ± 4	12 ± 1	52
	Acet[d]	20 ± 1	12 ± 1	61
	Acet + 4-MP	27 ± 3	14 ± 2	59
Fasted	Control	62 ± 6	9 ± 1	48
	Alc	20 ± 4	5 ± 1	5
	Alc + 4-MP	42 ± 8	11 ± 2	42
	Acet	50 ± 3	11 ± 1	49
	Acet + 4-MP	45 ± 3	15 ± 1	44

[a] Polysomes containing more than 3 ribosomes.
[b] Alc = ethanol 200 mg %.
[c] 4-MP = 4-methylpyrazole 1.5 mM.
[d] Acet = Acetaldehyde 2 mg %.
[e] All values are expressed as mean + SEM.

Carbon tetrachloride likewise rapidly destroys the endoplasmic reticulum, and lowers the rates of albumin synthesis, but as with ethanol, some of the effects can be ameliorated by enhanced amino acid supplementation (40). Both these toxic agents, ethanol and CCl_4, disrupt the subcellular mechanism for the synthesis of albumin and result in an acute loss in the albumin synthesizing capacity. However, the total potential is not destroyed, at least during the acute exposure, since significant recovery can be promoted rapidly by enhanced nutrition.

HEALTH AND DISEASE

Clinically, nutrition complicates so many diseases that, in vivo, it is difficult to clearly evaluate the effects of any perturbation in terms of albumin synthesis. This has been shown rather clearly in the observation made repeatedly in patients with cirrhosis of the liver, particularly in those patients whose disease is complicated by the development of ascites. Here, while the serum albumin level is depressed, the total exchangeable albumin pool is frequently normal or elevated. The rates of albumin synthesis in subjects remove from the toxic effects of ethanol and given adequate nutrition, were normal or elevated in 2/3 of the nineteen subjects studied (41).

The relation between nutrition and albumin synthesis is not based solely on amino acid supply. For example, protein losing enteropathy is a condition which may accompany any intestinal disorder characterized by mucosal weeping, lympathic obstruction, or specific intraluminal tumors such as gastric polyps. If the lesion which is spilling protein is high up in the GI tract, the resultant degraded peptides and amino acids should be delivered to the liver and albumin synthesis should increase, but this is not observed. It is as if the body recognizes the futility of increasing albumin synthesis only to have it destroyed. The hypoalbuminemia that develops is a complex end result of an eventual imbalance between the protein loss and the inability of the liver to synthesize increased quantities of albumin. In order to relieve the hypoalbuminemia it is necessary to correct the primary lesion within the intestinal tract.

The "wisdom of the body" does not always operate in a consistent manner. In the nephrotic syndrome large quantities of albumin are excreted as well as degraded by renal tubules. It would be expected that the futility of increasing the synthesis of albumin would be recognized. However, this is not the case. In rats made nephrotic with puromycin albumin synthesis was enhanced in perfused livers as well as in liver slices (42, 43). Rat liver microsomes isolated from rats made nephrotic with nephrotoxic serum also exhibited increased albumin synthesis (44). In studies on 30 adult nephrotics, the fractional rate of catabolism of albumin was increased in 19 patients, and the rate of albumin synthesis was increased in 11, with no patient having a synthetic rate less than normal (45).

COLLOID OSMOTIC PRESSURE

Sometimes the nature of regulation can be related to the biochemical's function. For example, a high level of energy in the form of ATP will act as a negative modulator of energy producing reactions. Likewise, serum albumin whose main function, aside from transport, is to maintain the colloid osmotic pressure of blood is also regulated by the serum's osmotic pressure.

The early work of Magnus Bjørneboe clearly demonstrated a reciprocal depression in serum albumin levels associated with a rise in globulin levels in patients with hepatitis (46). This observation has resulted in the eventual proof of the concept that alterations in colloid content probably at or near the site of albumin synthesis plays an important role in the regulation of

albumin production. In experimental situations, in which excessive endogenous globulin is synthesized associated with hyperimmunization, or
dextran or gammaglobulin is infused in vivo, the rate of albumin synthesis
decreases in an attempt to maintain effective colloid content. These studies
in vivo have been confirmed frequently in isolated perfused liver systems,
where excessive colloid content in the perfusate has inhibited the rates of
albumin synthesis as determined by the incorporation of precursors into de
novo synthesized albumin (47–50) (Table 5). The presence of Macrodex
dextran, mol.wt. 70,000) in an incubation medium containing liver slices
decreased the incorporation of radioactivity into albumin. When a cell
free system was tested the effect observed with the liver slice did not take
place. The integrity of the cell is necessary for oncotic pressure to effect
albumin synthesis (51).

In vivo, however, the depression in albumin synthesis seen in excessive
colloid states is more related to an increment in extra-vascular colloid
than in intravascular colloid content. In this regard, it is interesting to
note that whereas the plasma entering the liver and the lymph leaving the
liver have albumin contents which are closely approximated, the hepatic
interstitial space, 10% to 15% of wet liver weight, has an albumin content
one-tenth that of either the plasma or the lymph (52). Further, the liver,
a low pressure hydrostatic system, has a sinusoidal bed which offers very
little impediment to transport of molecules of up to 250,000 molecular
weight. This seeming paradox of an interstitial fluid with a very low albumin
content in equilibrium with two liver fluid components containing much
higher albumin levels which are in themselves in rapid equilibrium can
partially be explained by the observation that the hepatic interstitial
space is a complex protein polysaccharide matrix. This matrix has an
excluded volume which permits solubility of small molecules but which

Table 5. Effect of colloid on albumin synthesis

		In vivo
Colloid		*Change in albumin synthesis*
IgG	6.1%	−23%
Dextran	1.7%	−32%
		In vitro
Albumin	2.7%	0
Albumin	0.4–0.6%	+53%
Albumin	7%	−31%
Albumin	2.7% + 1% sucrose	−46%

will limit the solubility of other large molecules such as albumin (53–55). In any event, this suggests that the fluid bathing the liver cells, the site of albumin synthesis, contains a low colloid content, and this colloid content might prove a very effective and sensitive mechanism to effect a colloid osmotic regulation.

While these observations are true for substances other than albumin, excessive levels of serum albumin are prevented from accumulating in the plasma not by means of changes in albumin synthesis, but by increases in the rates of albumin degradation, as well as the spilling of significant quantities of albumin in the urine. As much as eighty percent of an infusion of albumin may be dissipated within one 24 hr. period under experimental situations (49). Thus, the continued infusion of albumin in an attempt to raise the serum albumin level without correcting the underlying disease entity is fraught with failure. It is of interest to note that osmotic regulation is not only an important consideration in man, but there is perhaps a parallel situation in the shark, which maintains equilibrium with its external environment by maintaining a urea concentration of 3–4000 mg/100 ml. As the shark is moved from salt water to fresh water, the concentration of urea drops and an albumin-like protein makes its appearance in the serum (56, 57).

ENVIRONMENT

Very few studies have been done about the effects of environment on the rates of albumin production. It is known that elevations in temperature either experimentally or in tropical climates will result in a depression in the serum albumin level as well as a lowering in the rate of albumin synthesis (58). Globulin levels are frequently elevated and the exact mechanism, therefore, between the changes in albumin levels or albumin synthesis and elevations in temperature are not clearly discernible. Increases in altitude have also been felt to be associated with changes in albumin degradation, but the effects on synthesis are not known (59, 60). As space travel and exploration becomes a more prevalent part of our changing world, it would be of importance to know something more about the effects of altered gravity on protein synthesis in general.

In summary, the effects of altered nutrition, hormones and ethanol can be traced, in part, to specific alterations in RNA metabolism and or amino acid supply, and or as yet undefined translational events. In any event, albumin synthesis can be partially or wholly restored by an enhanced amino acid supply and factors capable of causing bound polysome aggregation.

The specific areas of albumin biosynthesis affected by colloid osmotic pressure and environmental factors are, as yet, unknown. One can speculate in the case of osmotic pressure: since an intact cell membrane is necessary for an effect, and endoplasmic reticulum is contiguous with cell membrane, small changes in cell volume due to altered external colloid osmotic pressure may result in conformational changes of the endoplasmic reticulum. The change in the topology of this membrane, could in turn, alter sites for the binding of ribosomes and in this manner affect albumin synthesis. Changes in environmental temperature results in reciprocal changes in globulin and albumin levels suggesting osmotic transduction; changes in barometric pressure due to altitude likewise can mediate its effects via an osmotic mechanism.

Disease is a major inbalance in an organ's or body's biochemistry. This inbalance results in a complex interdigitation of nutritional, hormonal and neural effects all of which can alter albumin synthesis in a variety of ways.

REFERENCES

1. Quinn PS, Gamble M, Judah JD: Biosynthesis of serum albumin in rat liver. Isolation and probable structure of "proalbumin" from rat liver. Biochem J 146:389–393, 1975.
2. Urban J, Inglis AS, Edwards K, et al: Chemical evidence for the difference between albumins from microsomes and serum and a possible precursor-product relationship. Biochem Biophys Res Commun 61:444–451, 1974.
3. Peters T Jr., Serum Albumin: Recent progress in the understanding of its structure and biosynthesis. Clin Chem 23:5–12, 1977.
4. Strauss AW, Donohue AM, Bettett CD, et al: Rat liver preproalbumin: In vitro synthesis and partial amino acid sequence. Proc Natl Acad Sci, USA 74:1358–1362, 1977.
5. Blobel G, Dobberstein B: Transfer of proteins across membranes. I. Presence of proteolytically processed and unprocessed nascent immunoglobulin light chains on membrane bound ribosomes of murine myeloma. J Cell Biol 67:835–851, 1975.
6. Devillers-Thiery A, Kindt T, Scheele G, et al: Homology in amino terminal sequence of precursors to pancreatic secretory proteins. Proc Nat Acad Sci USA 72:5016–5020, 1975.
7. Munro HN, Waddington S, Begg DJ: Effect of protein intake on ribonucleic acid metabolism in liver cell nuclei of the rat. J Nutr 85:319–328, 1965.
8. Baliga BS, Pronczuli AW, Munro HN: Regulation of polysome aggregation in a cell free system through amino acid supply. J Mol Biol 34:199–218, 1968.
9. Rothschild MA, Oratz M, Mongelli J, et al: Effects of a short-term fast on albumin synthesis studied in vivo, in the perfused liver, and on amino acid incorporation by hepatic microsomes. J Clin Invest 47:2591–2599, 1968.

10. Rothschild MA, Oratz M, Mongelli J, et al: Amino acid regulation of albumin synthesis. J Nutr 98:395–403, 1969.

11. Enwonwu CO, Munro HN: Rate of RNA turnover in rat liver in relation to intake of protein. Arch Biochem Biophys 138: 532–539, 1970.

12. McGown E, Richardson AG, Henderson LM, et al: Effect of amino acids on ribosome aggregation and protein synthesis in perfused rat liver. J Nutr 103:109–116, 1973.

13. Blobel G, Potter VR: Studies on free and membrane bound ribosomes in rat liver. I. Distribution as related to total cellular RNA. J Mol Biol 26:279–292, 1967.

14. Rothschild MA, Oratz M, Schreiber SS: Alcohol, amino acids and albumin synthesis. Gastro 67:1200–1213, 1974.

15. Khawaja JA: Interactions of ribosomes and ribosomal sub-particles with endoplasmic reticulum membranes in vitro: effect of spermine and magnesium. Biochim Biophys Acta 254:117–128, 1971.

16. Khawaja JA: Influence of spermine on amino acid incorporation by free, bound and reattached ribosomes from rat liver. Acta Chem Scand 26:3450–3457, 1972.

17. Igarashi K, Yabuki M, Yoshioka, Y, et al: Mechanism of stimulation of polyphenylalanine synthesis by spermidine. Biochem Biophys Res Comm 75:163–171, 1977.

18. Rothschild MA, Bauman A, Yalow RS, et al: The effect of large doses of desiccated thyroid on the distribution and metabolism of albumin ^{131}I in euthyroid subjects. J Clin Invest 36:422–428, 1957.

19. Rothschild MA, Schreiber SS, Oratz M, et al: The effect of adrenocortical hormones on albumin metabolism studied with ^{131}I albumin. J Clin Invest 37:1229–1235, 1958.

20. Tata JE, Widnell, CC: Ribonucleic acid synthesis during the early action of thyroid hormones. Biochem J 98:604–620, 1966.

21. Widnell JR, Tata JR: Additive effects of thyroid hormone, growth hormone and testosterone on deoxyribonucleic acid polymerase in rat liver nuclei. Biochem J 98:621–629, 1966.

22. Cox RF, Mathias AP: Cytoplasmic effects of cortisol in liver. Biochem J 115:777–787, 1969.

23. Drews J, Braverman G: Alterations in the nature of ribonucleic acid synthesized in rat liver during regeneration and after cortisol administration. J Biol Chem 242:801–808, 1967.

24. Yatvin MB, Wannemacher RW Jr: Action of adrenal corticoids on protein metabolism in the thioracil-treated rat. Endocrinology 76:418–426, 1965.

25. Enwonwu CO, Munro HN: Changes in liver polyribosome patterns following administration of hydrocortisone and actinomycin D. Biochim Biophys Acta 238:264–276, 1971.

26. Agarwal MK, Hanoune J, Yu FL, et al: Studies on the effect of cortisone on rat liver transfer ribonucleic acid. Biochm J 8:4806–4813, 1969.

27. Silber RH, Porter CC: Nitrogen balance, liver protein repletion and body composition of cortisone treated rats. Endocrinology 52:518–525, 1953.

28. Kaplan SA, Shimizu CS: Free amino acid and amine concentrations in liver: effects of hydrocortisone and fasting. Am J Physiol 202:695–698, 1962.

29. Schmid W, Sekeris CE: Sequential stimulation of extranucleolar and nucleolar RNA synthesis in rat liver by cortisol. FEBS Lett 26:109–112, 1972.

30. Talwar GP, Gupta SL, Gros F: Effect of growth hormone on ribonucleic acid metabolism. 3 Nature and characteristics of nuclear subfractions stimulated by hormone treatment. Biochem J 91:565-572, 1964.

31. Tata JR, Williams-Ashman HG: Effects of growth hormone and triodothyronine on amino acid incorporation by microsomal subfractions from rat liver. Eur J Biochem 2:366–374, 1967.

32. Korner A: Regulation of the rate of synthesis of messenger ribonucleic acid by growth hormone. Biochem J 92:449–456, 1964.
33. Roy AK, Dowbenko DJ: Role of growth hormone in the multi-hormonal regulation of messenger RNA for α_{2u} globulin in the liver of hypophysectomized on the synthesis of rat liver albumin. Biochemistry 16:3918–3922, 1977.
34. Keller GH, Taylor JM: Effect of hypophysectomy on the synthesis of rat liver albumin. J Biol Chem 251:3768–3773, 1976.
35. Kernoff LM, Pimstone BL, Solomon J, et al: The effect of hypophysectomy and growth hormone replacement on albumin synthesis and catabolism in the rat. Biochem J 124:529–535, 1971.
36. Reaven EP, Peterson DT, Reaven GM. The effect of experimental diabetes mellitus and insulin replacement on hepatic ultrastructure and protein synthesis. J Clin Invest 52:248–262, 1973.
37. Baligno HF, Neuhaus OW: Effect of insulin on the injury stimulated synthesis of serum albumin in the rat. Life Sci 9 (11) 1039–1044, 1970.
38. Rubin E, Lieber CS: Alcohol induced hepatic injury in non-alcoholic volunteers. N Eng J Med 278:869–876, 1968.
39. Oratz M, Rothschild MA, Schreiber SS: Alcohol, amino acids and albumin synthesis. II. Alcohol inhibition of albumin synthesis reversed by arginine and spermine. Gastro 71:123–127, 1976.
40. Oratz M, Rothschild MA, Burks A, et al: The influence of amino acids and hepatotoxic agents on albumin synthesis, polysomal aggregation and RNA turnover. In: Protein Turnover, GEW Wolstenholme, M O'Conner (eds), Elsevier, Amsterdam, Ciba Foundation Symposium 9 (new series) 1963, pp 131–153.
41. Rothschild MA, Oratz M, Zimmon D, et al: Albumin synthesis in Cirrhotic subjects with ascites studied with Carbonate-^{14}C. J Clin Invest 48:344–355, 1969.
42. Katz J, Bonorris G, Okuyama S, et al: Albumin synthesis in perfused liver of normal and nephrotic rats. Am J Physiol 212:1255–1260, 1967.
43. Marsh JB, Drabkin DL: Metabolic channeling in experimental nephrosis. IV. Net synthesis of plasma albumin by liver slices from normal and nephrotic rats. J Biol Chem 230:1073–1081, 1958.
44. Marsh JB, Drabkin DL, Braun GA: Factors in the stimulation of protein synthesis by subcellular preparations from rat liver. J Biol Chem 241:4168–4174, 1966.
45. Jensen H, Rossing N, Anderson SB, et al: Albumin metabolism in the nephrotic syndrome in adults. Clin Sci 33:445–457, 1967.
46. Bjørneboe M: Studies on the serum proteins in hepatitis. I. The relation between serum albumin and serum globulin. Acta Med Scand 123:393–401, 1946.
47. Rothschild MA, Oratz M, Franklin EC, et al: The effect of Hypergammaglobulinemia on albumin metabolism in hyperimmunized rabbits studied with albumin I^{131}. J Clin Invest 41:1564–1571, 1962.
48. Oratz M: Oncotic pressure and albumin synthesis. In: Plasma Protein Metabolism, MA Rothschild, T Waldmann (eds), New York, Academic Press, 1970, pp 223–238.
49. Rothschild MA, Oratz M, Evans C, et al: Alterations in albumin metabolism after serum and albumin infusions. J Clin Invest 43:1874–1880, 1964.
50. Dich J, Hansen SE, Thieden HD: Effect of albumin concentration and colloid osmotic pressure on albumin synthesis in the perfused rat liver. Acta Physiol Scand 89:352–358, 1973.
51. Huberman A: The in vitro effect of colloid osmotic pressure on albumin biosynthesis in normal rat liver. Res Invest Clin 25: 321–326, 1973.
52. Rothschild MA, Oratz M, Evans CD, et al: Role of hepatic interstitial albumin in regulating albumin synthesis. Am J Physiol 210:57–62, 1966.
53. Ogston AG, Phelps CF: The partition of solutes between buffer solutions and solutions

containing hyaluronic acid. Biochem J 78–827–833, 1961.
54. Laurent TC, Ogston AG: The interaction between polysaccharides and other macro-molecules. IV. The osmotic pressure of mixtures of serum albumin and hyaluronic acid. Biochem J 89:249–253, 1963.
55. Shaw M: Interpretation of osmotic pressure in solutions of one and two nondiffusible components. Biophys J 16:43–57, 1976.
56. Goldstein L, Forster RP: Osmoregulation and urea metabolism in the little skate raja erinacea. Am J Physiol 220:742–746, 1971.
57. Rasmussen LE, Rasmussen RA: Comparative protein and enzyme profiles of the cerebro-spinal fluid, extradural fluid, nervous tissue, and sera of elasmobranchs. In: Sharks, Skates and Rays, PW Gilbert, RF Mathewson, DP Rall (eds), Baltimore, Johns Hopkins, 1967, pp 361–380.
58. Oratz M, Walker C, Schreiber SS, et al: Albumin and fibrinogen metabolism in heat and cold stressed rabbits. Am J Physiol 213:1341–1349, 1967.
59. Surks, MI: Metabolism of human serum albumin in man during acute exposure to high altitude (14,100 feet). J Clin Invest 45:1442–1451, 1966.
60. Schnakenberg DD, Krabill LF, Weiser PC: The anorexic effect of high altitude on weight gain, nitrogen retention and body composition of rats. J Nutr 101:787–796, 1971.

6. Distribution and degradation of albumin

S. Jarnum and K.B. Jensen

S. Jarnum and K.B. Jensen

INTRODUCTION

Studies of distribution and degradation of albumin became possible when Sterling in 1951 (1) introduced radioiodine-labeled albumin and showed that it could be used to determine the turnover rate of albumin in man. Time passed has seen the appearance of better preparations and more correct mathematical treatment of observed data, which means that, to day, we are able to measure the distribution and degradation of albumin with high accuracy in practically any patient with disturbed albumin metabolism.

METHODS

1. *Preparations*

All the observations reported below are based on studies with radioiodine-labeled proteins. In most cases simultaneous studies were made with two proteins labeled with ^{131}I and ^{125}I respectively, for instance ^{131}I-albumin and ^{125}I-IgG, which permits, under identical conditions, a comparison of degradation and distribution of two proteins which are very different in structure and metabolism. It is possible because the peak energies of the two isotopes are widely apart, thus allowing for the simultaneous determination of the isotopes in one sample.

A number of requirements concerning purity of the protein, gentle labeling procedure, blocking of thyroid radioiodide uptake by means of stable iodide given orally throughout the study must be fulfilled in such studies (Table 1).

Table 1. Requirements in studies with radioiodine-labeled proteins

---

1. Isolation of pure, undenatured protein
   Possible for: albumin, IgG, IgM, transferrin, fibrinogen
2. Gentle labeling procedure
3. ^{131}I-Protein behaves as unlabeled undenatured protein in the body
4. Thyroid uptake of ^{131}I blocked throughout the study by means of stable iodide (^{127}I)
5. Rapid excretion of the label
   $k = 1.5$ day^{-1} for iodide when renal function is normal and thyroid uptake is blocked.

---

2. Practical procedure

The practical procedure is common to all clinical turnover studies. A known amount of labeled protein is given intravenously. Blood is withdrawn after 10 min. (for determination of plasma volume and intravascular protein mass) and at daily intervals for the duration of the study, a few days up to several weeks, depending on the purpose of the study. Urine and, in patients with gastrointestinal disease, stools are collected in 24 hrs. specimens. A more precise method of determining the amount of ^{131}I excreted is to make use of a whole body counter (Fig. 1). Whole body counting has shown that even the most meticulous collection of secreta fails to account for five to ten per cent of the total excretion, probably due to some iodide excretion in sweat.

3. Degradation

The degradation or the rate of catabolism was determined in two independent ways: as a metabolic clearance or by means of the plasma disappearance curve of the labeled protein.

3.1. Metabolic clearance

The metabolic clearance is calculated from the daily excretion of radio-iodide in urine and the daily average plasma concentration of the labeled protein, a calculation which is analogous to many renal function tests (Fig. 2). If diarrhoea or gastrointestinal protein loss (proven or probable) is present, the iodine lost in the stools must also be measured. The metabolic clearance is determined daily for eight to ten days, and the average value is taken as the value closest to the true metabolic clearance (3).

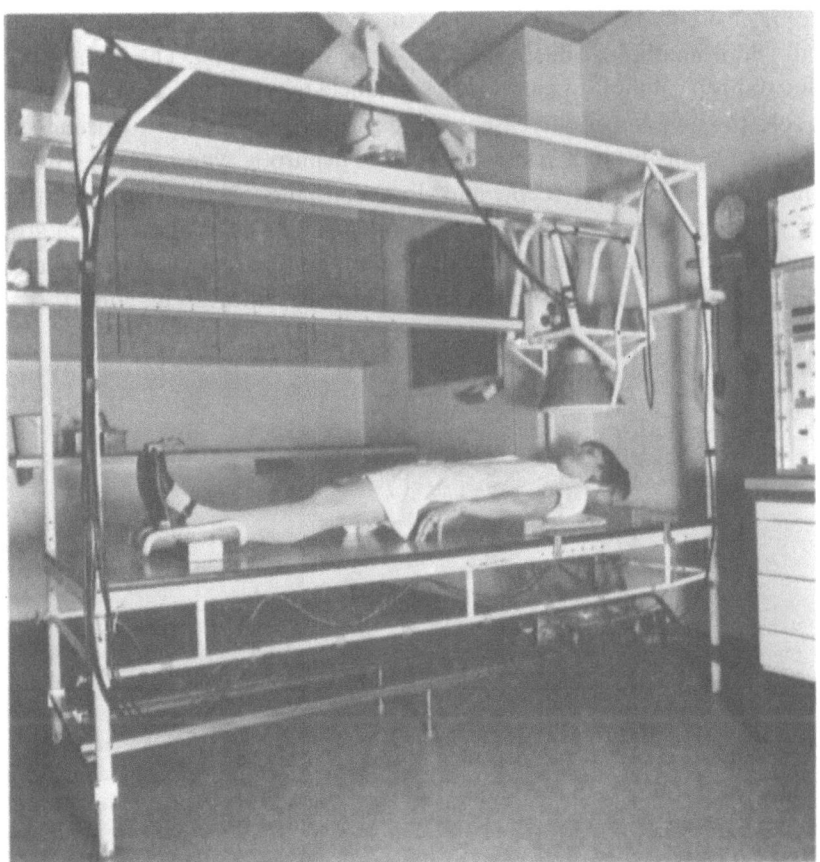

Fig. 1. Simple unshielded bed type whole body counter with two 3-inch NaI-Tl scintillation crystals, one above and one below the patient and each with a wide angle lead collimator. On counting they move from one end of the patient to the other in 5 to ten min. with constant speed.

3.2. *Analysis of plasma disappearance curve*

The plasma disappearance curve can be and has been treated mathematically in a number of ways. Because the labeled protein is injected into an open compartment i.e. the plasma pool and because degradation takes place in or close to the walls of the blood vessels, it can be shown that the degradation or fractional catabolic rate (FCR) is equal to the reciprocal of the integrated time-concentration area from time zero, i.e. the time of injection, to infinity (4, 5).

Fig. 3 shows the typical disappearance curve with an initial steep, curved fall and a final linear decrease in a semilogarithmic plot. The initial fall is due to both catabolism and transfer of labeled protein to the extravascular pools, the final linear decrease is due only to catabolism and abnormal loss if present, for instance proteinuria in the nephrotic syndrome. The figure shows the various intercepts and slope constants obtained by resolution of the plasma curve. They are used for a simple calculation of the area under the plasma curve ($_0\!\int^\infty Q_p \cdot dt$ where Q_p is the fraction of the injected dose of labeled protein present in the plasma or intravascular pool).

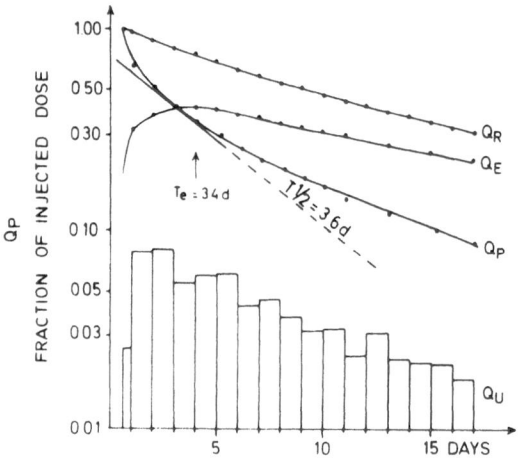

Fig. 2. Determination of metabolic clearance of a radioiodine-labeled plasma protein injected intravenously.

Q_U: The daily amount of radioiodine (fraction of injected dose) appearing in the urine. It represents radioiodide released during metabolic breakdown of the labeled protein.

Q_P : The amount of radioiodine-labeled protein present in the plasma (fraction of injected dose).

Q_U/Q_P: Daily clearance of labeled protein. Q_P denotes the mean concentration in the 24 hrs. period of urine collection. The average of 7–10 consecutive Q_U/Q_P is taken as the metabolic clearance.

Q_R: The amount of labeled protein (fraction of injected dose) remaining in the body (equal to $1 - Q_U$).

Q_E: Extravascular amount of labeled protein (equal to $Q_R - Q_P$).

D: Distribution = intravascular mass as fraction of total mass, can be roughly estimated from Q_P/Q_R at T_e, the time of "equilibrium", where Q_E attains maximum value and is horizontal. At this time protein of identical specific activity (cpm per mg protein) leaves and reenters the intravascular compartment (2).

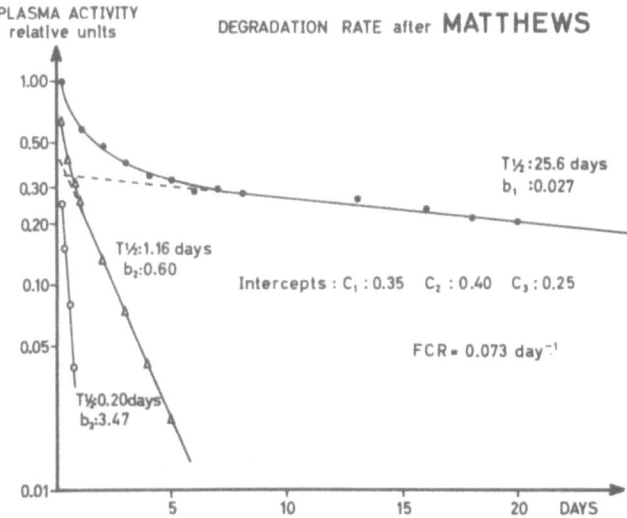

Fig. 3. Determination of fractional catabolic rate (FCR) by mathematical analysis of the plasma activity curve (fraction of injected dose of labeled protein remaining in the plasma). The curve is solved in two or three exponential functions each defined by its intercept with the y-axis (c) and its slope constant (b).
  FCR is calculated as:

$$(c_1/b_1 + c_2/b_2 + c_3/b_3)^{-1} \cdot day^{-1} \quad (4).$$

Total body activity determined by whole body counting follows a similar curve, but the final slope which is identical to that of the plasma curve, is attained at a much earlier time, which makes possible the conclusion of the study within a week (Fig. 4).

4. Distribution

Distribution which is here – for practical reasons – defined as the fraction or percentage of the total albumin pool which is located in the intravascular bed depends on the exchange rates between the intra- and extravascular pools of masses:

$$IVM \cdot k_{ie} = EVM \cdot k_{ei} \text{ g/day}$$

where: IVM = intravascular mass of albuming (g)
     k_{ie} = fraction of IVM transferred to EVM per day

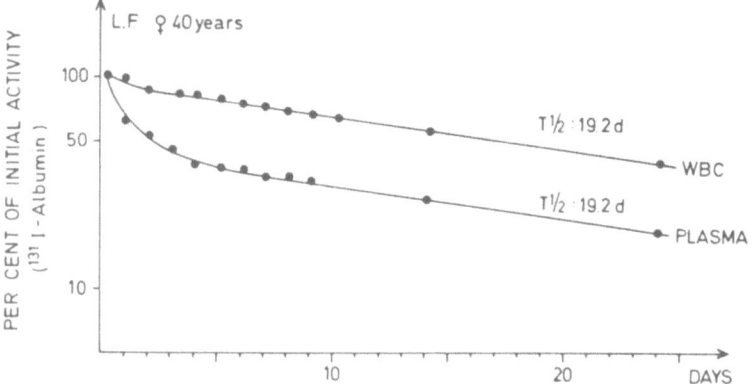

Fig. 4. Whole body activity curve (WBC) compared with plasma activity curve over more than three weeks. The final slopes are identical. Only whole body counting yields the final slope within a week.

and: EVM = extravascular mass of albumin (g)
         k_{ei} = fraction of EVM returned to IVM per day

   The equation is an oversimplification since, actually, a great number of extravascular pools exists (e.g. subcutaneous interstitial fluid, fluid of serous cavities, lymph in lymphatic vessels and nodules) with different return rates of albumin to the blood. However, the equation illustrates how EVM may increase either by an increase of k_{ie} (i.e. increased capillary permeability of the protein) or by a decrease of k_{ei} (e.g. in lymphatic obstruction).

   4.1 Distribution can be determined by three independent methods. One is the equilibrium time method (Fig. 2) (3) which is theoretically correct but rather inaccurate.

   4.2 From the plasma curve one obtains the distribution from:

$$D = \frac{\left(\dfrac{c_1}{b_1} + \dfrac{c_2}{b_2} + \dfrac{c_3}{b_3}\right)^2}{\dfrac{c_1}{b_1^2} + \dfrac{c_2}{b_2^2} + \dfrac{c_3}{b_3^2}}$$

where c's and b's are the various intercepts and slope constants obtained by resolution of the plasma curve (Fig. 3) (4).

4.3 Finally, one may calculate the distribution rate from the ratio between the integrated area under the plasma curve and that under the curve of the rest activity of the body determined by whole body counting (5).

NORMAL VALUES

Normal values of degradation and distribution of albumin in adults and children have been established by Rossing (6) and Krasilnikoff (7). They are shown in Table 2.

In adults the degradation or catabolic rate is about 9% of the intravascular albumin mass per day and the distribution 43%, which means that more than half the total albumin pool is located as extravascular albumin.

Compared to other major plasma proteins (Table 3) the FCR is low like that of IgG, and distribution is similar to that of transferrin with almost identical molecular weight.

Table 2. Normal degradation and distribution of albumin

	FCR, per cent per day	D, per cent
Children, 0–3 months	16.7 (10.9–22.5)*	35 (27–43)
Children, 3 months–2 years	10.8 (8.2–13.4)	45 (37–53)
Children, 2–5 years	9.2 (5.8–12.6)	48 (40–56)
Children, > 5 years	8.4 (6.0–10.8)	49 (43–55)
Adults	8.5 (6.5–10.5)	43 (35–51)

FCR = Fractional Catabolic Rate = degradation = percentage of IVM degraded per day
D = Distribution ratio = IVM as percentage of total albumin mass
*range – mean ± 2S.D.
Compilated from Krasilnikoff (7) and Rossing (6).

Table 3. Degradation and distribution of some plasma proteins

Plasma protein	Serum concentration g/l	Fractional catabolic rate % of intravasc. mass (IVM)/day	Synthetic rate g/175 cm/day	Molecular weight	Distribution ratio IVM as % of total mass
Albumin	42 (10%)	9 (9%)	11 (16%)	68,000	45 (8%)
Transf	2.2 (8%)	17 (7%)	1.1 (21%)	70,000	49 (5%)
IgG	11 (17%)	7 (21%)	2.1 (28%)	160,000	58 (12%)
IgM	0.8 (35%)	11 (14%)	0.3 (41%)	900,000	74 (15%)
Fibrinogen	3.6	25	2.2	360,000	84

In parenthesis: coefficient of variation

The coefficient of variation of serum concentration, catabolic rate and distribution of albumin is low compared to that of the immunoglobulins, which probably has the simple explanation that the exposure to antigens varies widely from person to person whereas everybody has to muster the same oncotic pressure by means of albumin to counterbalance the force of gravity.

DEGRADATION AND DISTRIBUTION OF ALBUMIN IN DISEASE

1. *Decreased degradation* (low FCR)

A low serum albumin may be associated with both decreased and increased catabolism. Table 4 shows diseases with decreased serum albumin and low degradation rates. In these diseases the synthesis rate of albumin is reduced. In the very rare congential condition, analbuminaemia, serum albumin is absent or present only in traces. The degradation of intravenously injected ^{131}I-albumin is very slow and a high fraction of the small albumin pool is located in the intravascular pool (8).

In cirrhosis of the liver the degradation (FCR) can be significantly decreased (9), the synthesis rate can also be about reduced, whereas distribution is only slightly less than normal. In patients with large ascites the distribution is low due to accumulation of extravascular albumin in the ascitic fluid (Fig. 5).

In malnourished patients (postgastrectomy and stagnant loop syndrome) the same pattern is present (Fig. 6). Their distribution is normal.

2. *Increased degradation*

Hypoalbuminaemia due to increased degradation is seen in true endogenous hypercatabolism and in abnormal protein loss (Table 5).

A true endogenous hypercatabolism of albumin is present in thyreo-

Table 4. Diseases with decreased albumin degradation (low FCR)

1.1. Analbuminaemia	– low synthesis
1.2. Cirrhosis of the liver	– low synthesis
1.3. Malnutrition	– low synthesis

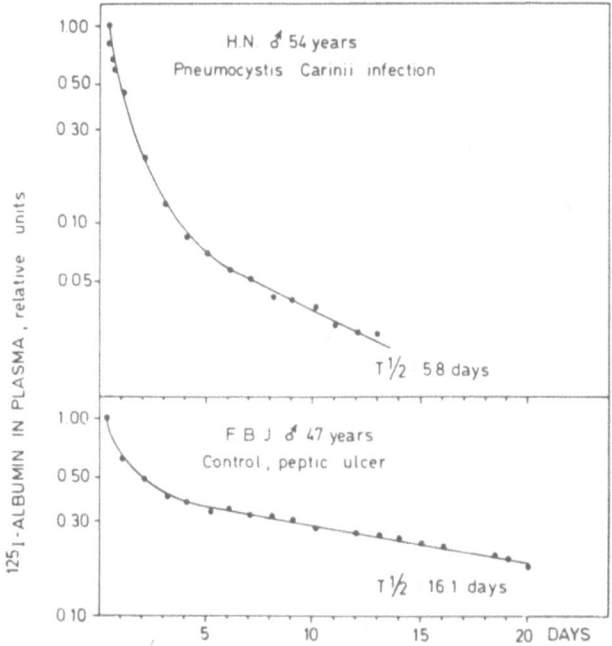

Fig. 7. ^{125}I-Albumin in plasma following intravenous injection in a patient with severe hypoalbuminaemia (serum albumin 4 g/l) and generalized pneumocystis carinii infection and in a control subject (lower half) studied with the same preparation.

In gastrointestinal disease an abnormal protein loss occurs in a great variety of diseases in all parts of the gastrointestinal tract (Table 5).

In Ménétrier's disease (= giant hypertrophic gastritis) the protein loss may be so severe that total or subtotal gastrectomy is required but, usually, it is mild or moderate.

In small intestinal disease intestinal lymphangiectasia due to congenital malformations of the lymphatic system may lead to the greatest protein loss seen, above all in infants where the disease carries a rather high lethality. Non-tropical sprue is regularly, but in no way always, associated with protein loss when untreated.

The same holds true for a number of neoplastic diseases: gastric cancer, carcinoma of the colon, polyposis (11).

In chronic inflammatory bowel disease an abnormal protein loss is almost a consistent finding. The degree of serum albumin depression is a good marker of disease activity, in particular in ulcerative colitis (12). The

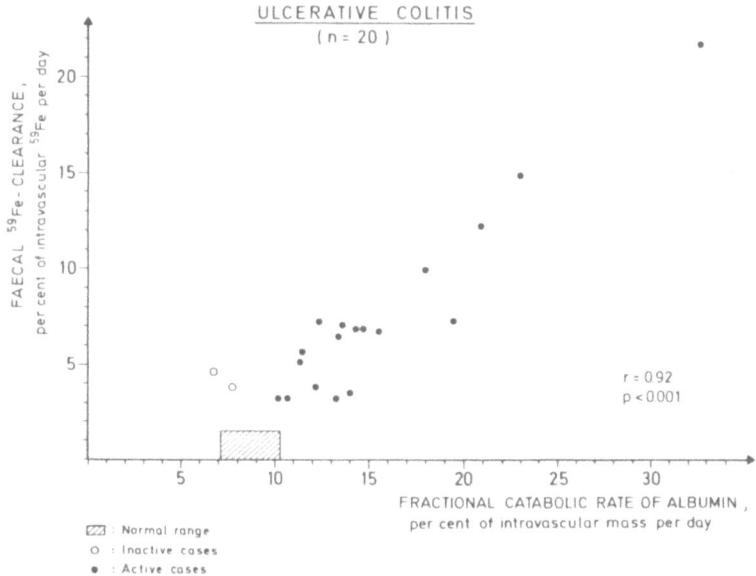

Fig. 8. Correlation between albumin degradation (FCR, x-axis) and intestinal ⁵⁹Fe-clearance following intravenous injection of ⁵⁹Fe-labeled iron dextran (y-axis) in 20 cases of ulcerative colitis (13).

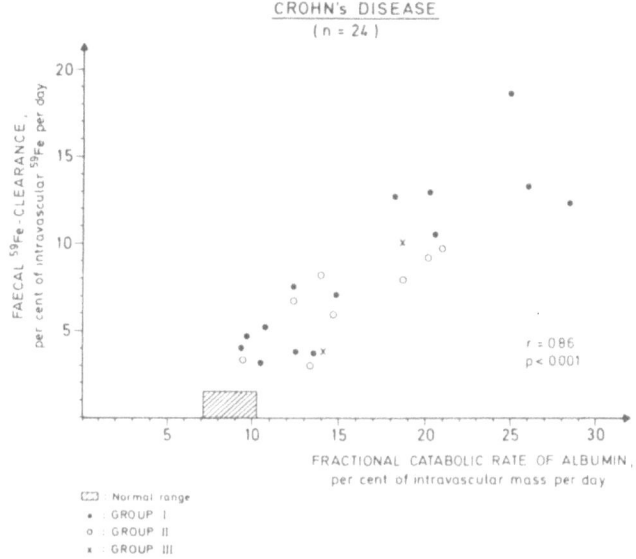

Fig. 9. Correlation between albumin degradation and intestinal ⁵⁹Fe-clearance (as in Fig. 8) in 24 cases of Crohn's disease. The diagnosis rests on microscopy of surgically removed intestinal segments in every case (13).

low serum albumin is the result of increased degradation due to abnormal protein loss (Figs. 8 and 9) (13).

In the nephrotic syndrome a selective protein loss is present with preferential glomerular loss of smaller protein molecules. Therefore, the increase of albumin catabolism is significantly higher than that of for instance IgG with a molecular weight more than twice as high. In contrast, gastro-

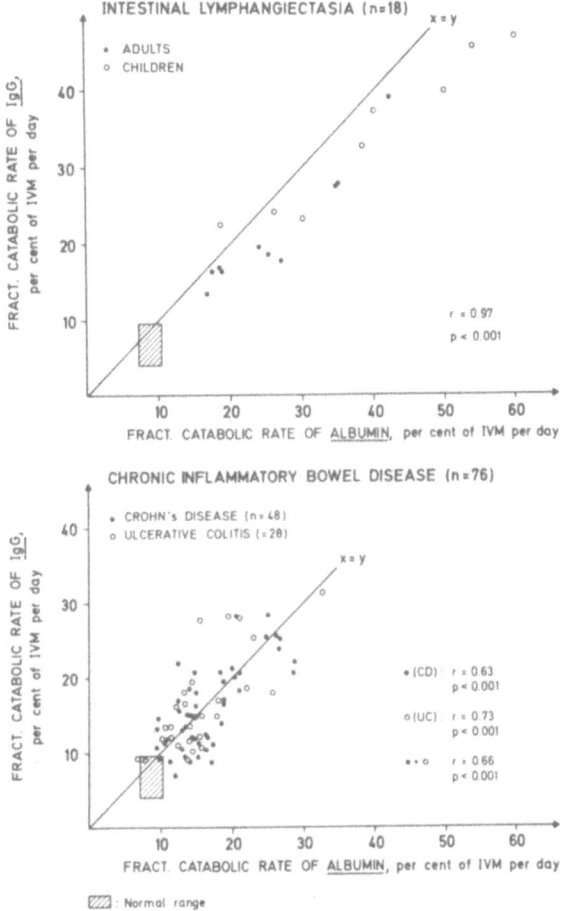

Fig. 10. Fractional catabolic rate of albumin and IgG determined in simultaneous studies with ^{131}I-albumin and ^{125}I-IgG in 76 patients with chronic inflammatory bowel disease (lower part) and in 18 patients with intestinal lymphangiectasia (upper part).

The line of identity (x = y) is drawn.

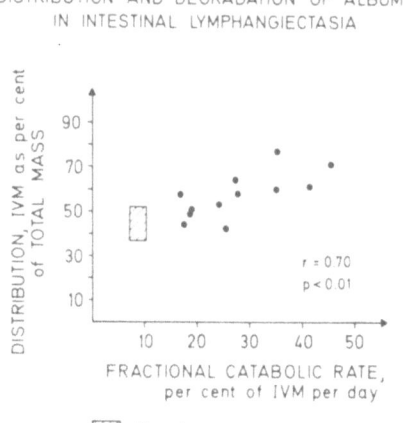

Fig. 11. Correlation between fractional catabolic rate and distribution ratio of albumin in 12 patients with intestinal lymphangiectasia.

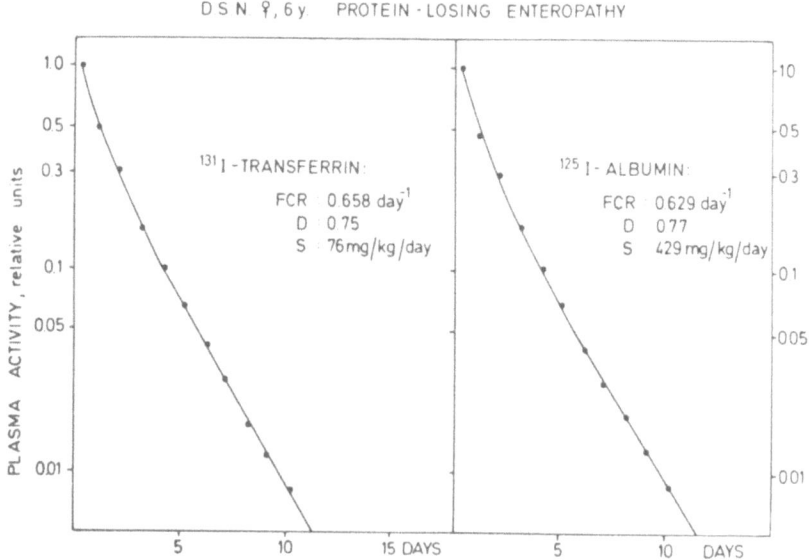

Fig. 12. ^{131}I-albumin and ^{125}I-transferrin plasma disappearance curves following intravenous injection to a six year old child (D.S.N.) with severe protein-losing enteropathy due to intestinal lymphangiectasia.

intestinal protein loss is considered a "bulk loss" which hits all circulating proteins to the same extent.

In simultaneous studies with labeled albumin and IgG we found this to be the case in chronic inflammatory bowel disease (Fig. 10, lower part), since there was a similar increase of the fractional catabolic rate of the two proteins. However, in intestinal lymphangiectasia (Fig. 10, upper part) the increase of IgG degradation was less than that of albumin which suggests a preferential loss of the smaller albumin molecules in this essentially non-inflammatory condition.

3. Distribution

Distribution ratio of albumin is low when large extravascular accumulations of albumin are present, for instance in cirrhotic patients with ascites, which usually has a high protein concentration. Protein concentration is also high in oedema fluid in lymphatic obstruction.

In hypoproteinaemic oedema, for instance in the nephrotic syndrome or in protein-losing enteropathy, the distribution ratio is normal or even high in agreement with the fact that the albumin concentration of oedema fluid is often extremely low.

We have tried to establish whether a correlation exists between distribution and degradation of albumin. In normal persons we found no correlation to be present. Neither did we find a correlation in the nephrotic syndrome or in chronic inflammatory bowel disease. However, in intestinal lymphangiectasia (Fig. 11) we found a positive and statistically significant correlation between fractional catabolic rate of albumin and the distribution ratio ($r = 0.70$, $p < 0.01$). It suggests that capillary permeability is decreased in this condition which may be related to the fact that these patients almost invariably present with a high haematocrit and a low blood volume.

A typical ^{131}I-albumin and ^{125}I-transferrin plasma disappearance curve in a child with intestinal lymphangiectasia is shown in Fig. 12. The curve is almost monoexponential which means that a very high fraction of the total pool is circulating in the plasma.

ACKNOWLEDGEMENTS

The work was supported by grants from P. Carl Petersens Fond and Christian d. X's Fond.

REFERENCES

1. Sterling K: The turnover rate of serum albumin in man as measured by I[131]-tagged albumin. J clin Invest 30:1228–1237, 1951.
2. Pearson JD, Veall N, Vetter H: A practical method for plasma albumin turnover. In: Radioakt Isotop Klin Forsch, vol III, Urban & Schwarzenberg, München & Berlin, 1958, p 290.
3. Campbell RM, Cuthbertson DP, Matthews CM, McFarlane AS: Behaviour of [14]C- and ^{131}I-labelled plasma proteins in the rat. Int J appl Radiat Isotopes 1:66–84, 1956.
4. Matthews CME: The theory of tracer experiments with ^{131}I-labelled plasma proteins. Phys med Biol 2:36–53, 1957.
5. Nosslin B: Applications of tracer theory to protein turnover studies. J nucl biol Med 9:18–19, 1966.
6. Rossing N: Human albumin metabolism determined with radioiodinated albumin, Munksgaard, Copenhagen, 1971 (Thesis.)
7. Krasilnikoff PA: Albumin metabolism in normal mature and premature children, FADL's Forlag, Copenhagen, 1975. (Thesis.)
8. Bennhold H, Kallee E: Comparative studies on the half-life of ^{131}I-labeled albumins and non-radioactive human serum albumin in a case of analbuminaemia. J clin Invest 38:863, 1959.
9. Hasch E, Jarnum S, Tygstrup N: Albumin metabolism as a liver function test in cirrhosis. In: Liver Research, St. Catherine Press, Ltd., Bruges, Belgium, 1967, p 453–458.
10. Jensen H, Rossing N, Andersen SB, Jarnum S: Albumin metabolism in the nephrotic syndrome in adults. Clin Sci 33:445–457, 1967.
11. Jarnum S: Protein-Losing Gastroenteropathy, Blackwell Scientific Publications, Oxford, 1963.
12. Jensen KB, Jarnum S, Koudahl G, Kristensen M: Serum orosomucoid in ulcerative colitis. Its relation to clinical activity, protein loss and turnover of albumin and IgG. Scand J Gastroent 11:177–183, 1976.
13. Jarnum S, Jensen KB: Fecal radioiodide excretion following intravenous injection of ^{131}I-albumin and ^{125}I-immunoglobulin G in chronic inflammatory bowel disease. Gastroenterology 68:1433–1444, 1975.

7. Serum albumin in clinical practice: A historical review

C. L. H. MAJOOR

Since it is impossible to survey in a few pages all important facts that have been ascertained and all conclusions that have been reached during the last 60 years, on the significance of serum albumin metabolism for the symptomatology, the course and the treatment of many frequently occurring internal diseases and their complications, I shall restrict myself in this review to those clinical and experimental facts, which have impressed me most during almost 40 years of interest in this field of medicine.

The story really started in 1895, with the classical study by the physiologist Ernest H. Starling "On the absorption of fluids from the connective tissue spaces" (1). The most important conclusions of this paper are still worth to be reprinted:

1. "Salt solutions, isotonic with the blood-plasma, can be and are absorbed directly by the blood vessels. This statement probably holds good for dropsical fluids containing small percentages of proteids."
2. "A backward filtration into the vessels is mechanically impossible in the connective tissues of the limbs, of the muscles and of the glands similar in structure to the sub-maxillary."
3. "The proteids of serum have an osmotic pressure of about 30 mm to 40 mm Hg. Absorption of isotonic salt solutions by the blood vessels is determined by this osmotic pressure of the serum proteids."
4. "The proteids of the tissue fluids, when not used in the tissues themselves, are probably absorbed mainly, if not exclusively, by the lymphatic system."

It has lasted however up till 1917, before the clinician A.A. Epstein had applied Starling's concept to explain the edema of patients with the nephrotic syndrome. As can be seen in Table 1, Epstein (2) found extremely low albumin- and almost normal globulin-levels in sera from patients with

Table 1. Data from Albert A. Epstein, 1917 (2)

Average composition of blood sera, g/l				
	Total protein	Globulin	Albumin	Cholesterol
Normal	74	27	47	±1.5
Cardiac conditions	64	22	44	1.6
Chronic parenchymatous nephritis	39	35	4.7	5.6
Average composition of effusion fluids, g/l:				
Cardiac conditions	34	12	18	
Chronic parenchymatous nephritis	2.9	2.9	0	
Edema fluid, g/l:				
Chronic parenchymatous nephritis	0.1	0.08	0.02	

chronic parenchymatous nephritis. In contradistinction to the findings in patients with cardiac disease, almost no protein, and particularly no albumin, was detected in serous effusions and edema fluid of patients with the nephrotic syndrome. The increased level of serum cholesterol in patients with this syndrome was, as shown in Epstein's data, already known 60 years ago. However, the technique employed to separate albumin from globulins was not indicated. The method of half saturation with $(NH_4)_2SO_4$ was probably used.

In the same year, 1917, when Epstein published his study, the famine edema of the first World War had reached its culminating point in Austria and Germany. Two excellent publications about this syndrome by Jansen, from the Second Department of Medicine of Munich University, deserve to be mentioned (3). Apart from a thorough description of the clinical entity of this syndrome with its weakness, depression, emaciation, edema of the face and the lower extremities, moderate anemia, bradycardia, low blood-pressure and abundant polyuria, Jansen performed a careful balance study in 7 male patients with edema from a nursing home (group A) and four prisoners (group B). During these experiments dietary intake was standardized with the utmost care and controlled meticulously. The quantity and quality of food and fluid intakes were the same as the rations patients received during the preceding months. The mean intake of the first 7 patients studied (group A) amounted to 1126 calories, two liters of liquid and 40–65 g of protein. The mean nitrogen balance per day was 3.4 g negative. The subjects of group B had performed field work during the period preceding the experimental week. During the experiment they were kept indoors. The mean intake was 1760 calories, more than 3.5 liters of water and 80–115 g of protein, mainly from animal origin. Notwithstanding the high intake of protein and the change of moderate work to relative rest during the experiment, the nitrogen balance of these prisoners was still negative with a mean of 0.14 g per day.

The total serum protein, as determined by Kjeldahlometric method, was between 40.3 and 73 g/l in group A and between 58 and 65 g/l in the subjects of group B (normal range in Jansen's laboratory: 65–85 g/l). However albumin was not measured in any of these patients.

It is important to note that Jansen in 1917, while doing his experiments, established that in the healthy Bavarian population without edema, urinary salt excretion, measured as Cl^- by Volhard's method, was relatively high, amounting to 20 to even 45 g per day. The diet used in his study in both group A and B, contained 35–45 g of salt.

To determine the impact of high salt intakes in the war-rations of 1917 on the pathogenesis of famine edema, Jansen performed another accurate balance study in a 54 year old woman with a stricture of the esophagus due to carcinoma, that in the course of 3 years had seriously interfered with normal food intake. Her bodyweight had dropped from 65 to 34 kg (almost 50%). However edema did not occur. During the study, the patient received milk, butter and cakes (almost 1100 calories). The salt intake was low: 2 g per day. As can be seen in Fig. 1 the consequences of two water loads and one water and salt load were studied. During both waterloads, it is evident that diuresis was rapid and complete. However bodyweight showed a slight fall with a moderately negative NaCl balance. In the salt load period, from the 8th to the 20th day of the experiment, 30 g of extra salt per day – or the mean NaCl content of war-rations in 1917 – were given. 82 g of NaCl were retained in the first 9 days, bodyweight rose from 34 to 40 kg and for the first time of patient's illness, edema appeared, first at the eyes, subsequently in the face, the feet and the arms. On the 9th day body weight started to fall and an "escape fenomenon" occurred, as has been shown by modern investigators, e.g. during long lasting aldosterone-administration. It is important to be mentioned that hemoglobin and dry weight of blood decreased in this period of salt loading. The reduction of these values amounted to 20–25% and suggests that there was a rise in plasma-volume of some 500 ml.

Finally, Jansen has also studied the effect of addition of 135 g of butter (1100 calories) per day for 6 days to one of his patients from group B with

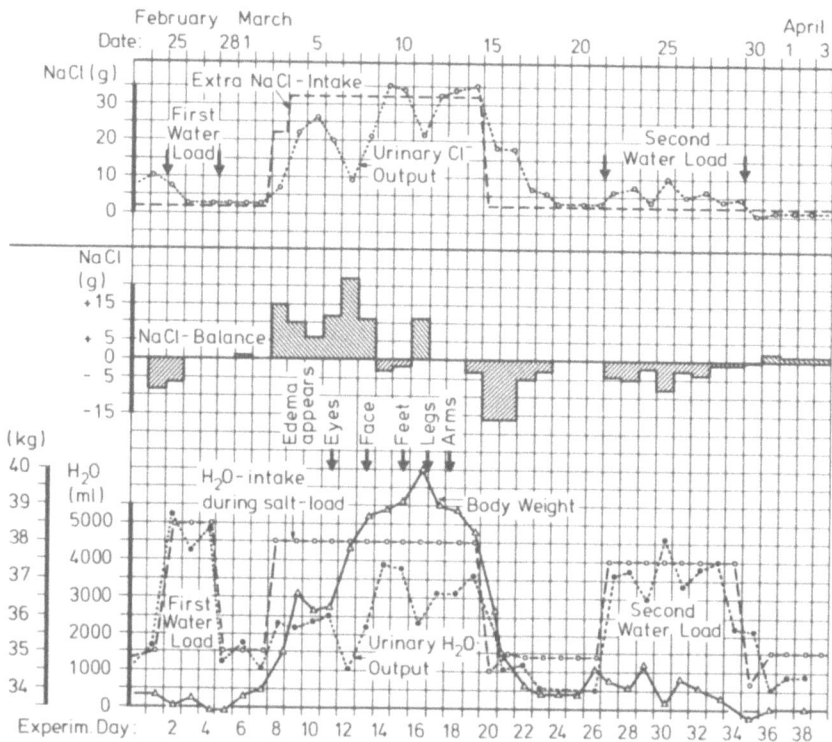

Fig. 1. NaCl-balance study during water, and NaCl with water loads in a 54 year old female with extreme emaciation, caused by a stenosing carcinoma of the oesophagus. (Adapted from: WH Jansen (1920) (3).)

famine edema. A second subject from this group received 200 g of extra sugar per day (800 calories). In both patients the nitrogen balance became immediately positive, with a mean of 3.26 g of nitrogen per day (about 20 g of protein) in the man who received extra butter and a mean of 15.3 g of protein per day in the case of sugar supplementation. Concomitant with these findings the salt balance became negative in both patients and after 6 days of supplementary feeding, their body weight had fallen more than 4 kg.

The main conclusions that can be drawn from these studies by now 60 year old, are:

1. In famine periods a sufficient intake of protein cannot ensure the nitrogen balance when the total caloric intake is insufficient.

2. Inanition does cause an "edema tendency" that only leads to overt clinical edema if the diet contains ample salt.
3. The negative nitrogen balance on low caloric diets could be reversed immediately by addition of 135 g of butter or 200 g of sugar. This reversal of nitrogen balance went hand in hand with a negative chloride balance and a loss of body weight of more than 4 kg in only 6 days.

So the finding of a protein sparing effect of glucose during fasting, regularly attributed in American literature (4) to Gamble, and discussed in his well known lecture syllabus from 1947 (5), has already definitely been made 30 years earlier by Jansen in his meticulous clinical work.

After Howe in 1921 (6, 7) had proposed sodium sulfate (21.5 g%) for the separation of serum globulins from albumin and Govaerts in 1927 (8) had derived a relatively simple formula to calculate the colloid osmotic pressure of serum, based on these albumin and globulin contents, the determination of serum albumin levels became popular in many clinics all over the world as a useful tool to judge blood and body hydration in severely ill patients. Especially John P. Peters and his coworkers from Yale University have drawn attention to the fact that serum albumin is not only low in patients with the nephrotic syndrome, as Epstein had established earlier, but also in other clinical conditions, such as: severe infections and heart failure. Peters and Eisenman stated in 1933 (9, p. 810): "The function of the serum proteins which will be the chief concern of this paper is the protein osmotic pressure and its relation to the theory of transudation and edema formation proposed by Starling". The authors concluded that "edema may be expected to appear in non-nephritic cases when serum albumin falls to about 3%" (p. 829). However three restrictions were made:

Firstly the authors considered a "well-recognized fact that by a high salt and fluid intake edema can be produced at a protein level higher than that at which it is likely to occur spontaneously" (p. 818). Secondly: "Anemia increases the tendency to edema and raises the albumin and the osmotic pressure at which it may be expected to 4% and 26 mm Hg respectively" (p. 830). And thirdly: "The critical level for edema production, 3%, applies only to malnutrition edema. It is distinctly above the similar level . . . found in the nephrotic syndrome" (p. 831).

In Chapter II of Peters' well known monograph "Body Water, the exchange of fluids in man" (10), he has also paid attention to other factors that may influence edema formation, for example: tissue tension and drainage by the lymphatics. He quoted Landis's studies (11, 12) and suggested that insufficient oxygenation of blood may permit proteins to escape freely from capillaries. I feel that this, probably important, factor is somewhat neglected in modern thinking about edema formation.

Meanwhile in many research institutes investigations were carried out to ascertain the effect of diets deficient in protein and/or calories, on the level of hemoglobin, hematocrit and albumin and on total nitrogen balance. From one of these studies, that has impressed me many years ago, I would like to review a few data. Weech, Goettsch and coworkers from the Department of Pediatrics, Columbia University, New York, have studied the effect of extremely protein deficient diets with adequate calories on erythrocytes and hemoglobin in dogs (13). Because of inanition the diets were not always completely consumed by the animals, so that a moderate caloric restriction certainly has played a role during the later weeks of the experiments. As shown in Fig. 2, during 80 days of experiment, the

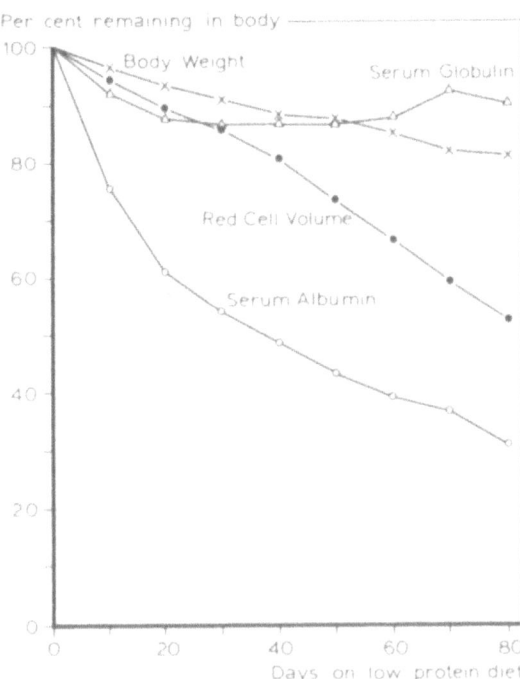

Fig. 2. Losses in the circulating proteins during 80 days on low protein diets, expressed as percentages of the original amount, remaining after various time intervals. Compilation of results of two large series of experiments in dogs. (Adapted from: AA Weech et al. (1937) (13) with permission from the editor.)

mean relative decrease of circulating albumin amounted to 70% and was larger than the fall of red cell volume, while body weight decreased only 20%, partly because of the occurrence of hypo-proteinemic edema. When the losses of protein from total body and from the blood were calculated (Fig. 3), it was found that albumin loss amounted to only 3.1% and loss of tissue protein contributed almost 80% of the total nitrogen loss. So, although albumin proved to be the most sensitive marker of nitrogen loss as a result of a protein deficient diet, the absolute loss of hemoglobin was 6 times and the loss of tissue protein was 25 times greater than that of albumin. As the diets in these experiments were similar in composition to those of children with Kwashiorkor, I feel that these, now 40 year old experiments, have still a distinct meaning for present medical thinking. Another important point made by Weech and his collaborators was that Starling's concept of fluid movement to and from the extracellular fluid, not only explains a tendency towards edema formation in hypoalbumin-

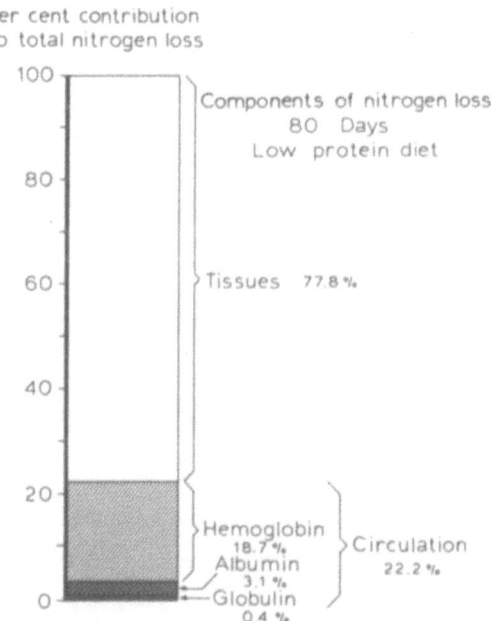

Fig. 3. Relationship between the total loss of protein from the body and the losses in the circulating proteins after 80 days on a low protein diet. Compilation of results from several series of experiments in dogs.
(Adapted from: AA Weech et al. (1937) (13) with permission from the editor.)

emia, as a result of a decreased colloid osmotic pressure, but also requires a reduction of plasma volume. That this occurred in the dogs studied by Weech et al., is demonstrated in Fig. 4. It is, however, interesting to note that the fall of red cell volume and of blood volume was distinctly greater that that of plasma volume. The authors quoted the studies of Darrow and Buckman, who, as early as 1928 (14), found low plasma and blood volumes in nephrotic children, and, what is even more important to mention in this regard: Chang's work from Peiping Union Medical College, in 1932 (15). Besides the low blood volume in patients with nephrosis during the edematous phase, he found a low blood volume and a low total plasma protein concentration in 7 patients with famine edema. These two parameters were normalized during recovery, as can be seen in Fig. 5, composed from Chang's data.

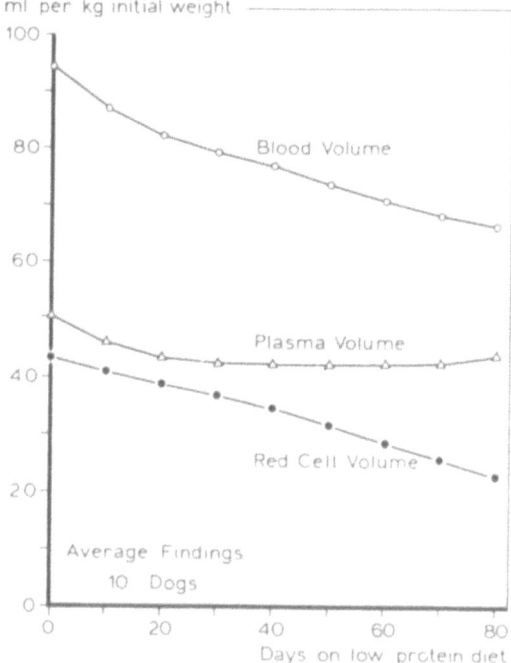

Fig. 4. Changes in blood volume, plasma volume and red cell volume during 80 days on a low protein diet in ml per kg initial body weight. Compilation of results from 60 experiments in dogs.
(Adapted from: AA Weech et al. (1937) (13) with permission from the editor.)

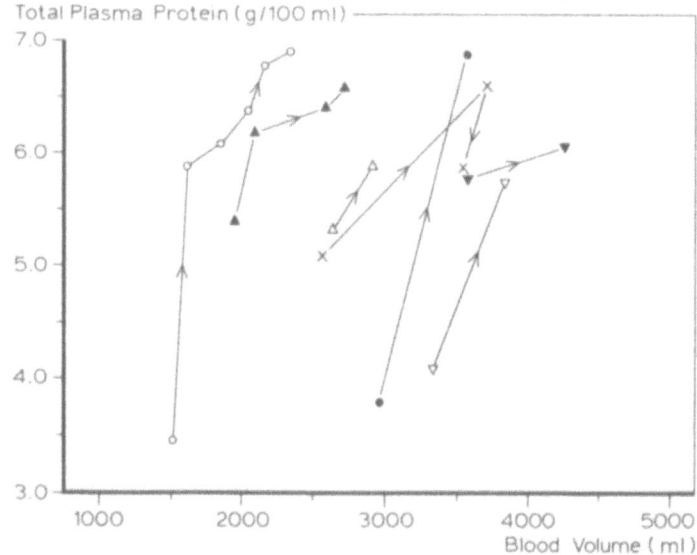

Fig. 5. Relationship between total plasma protein and blood volume (CO-method) in 7 subjects with nutritional edema. At the beginning of the observation period, blood volume was lower than the normal standard. Both parameters rose during the recovery phase towards the normal range.
(Composed from data from HC Chang (1932) (15).)

In June 1939, Borst from Amsterdam started a study on the frequency of hypoalbuminemia in hospitalized patients. In the course of two years, serum albumin, measured according to the method as described by Howe (7), was estimated in 614 patients with all types of internal diseases. A moderate number of severely ill surgical patients, seen in consultation, was included in this study. Severe hypoalbuminemia with a serum albumin concentration below 30 g/l was found in 94 patients, moderate hypoalbuminemia (30–35 g/l) was established in 102 patients. As shown in Table 2 (16) the highest percentage of severe to moderate hypoalbuminemia was found in patients with pneumococcal pneumonia with or without empyema, a disease that has almost disappeared at the present time from medical wards. Other serious infections by common bacteria showed a comparable high score. In active lungtuberculosis, notwithstanding a hectic fever in many of these patients, the frequency of severe hypoalbuminemia was relatively much lower. A similar finding was also shown by Peters and Eisenman (9). In severe trauma and war casualties, a low

Table 2. Frequency of severe hypoalbuminemia in selected patients admitted in the "Binnengasthuis" Amsterdam 1939–1941

	Number of patients	Serum albumin concentration (g/l)			per cent of total < 35 g/l
		> 35	30–35	< 30	
Tuberculous infections with moderate clinical activity	17	15	2	0	12%
Active tuberculosis of lungs	12	8	2	2	33%
Pneumonia with or without empyema	37	9	13	11	65%
Other serious infections	45	15	10	20	66%
Severe trauma and war casualties	15	11	3	1	27%
Ulcerative colitis	15	10	2	3	33%
Heart failure	70	45	17	8	36%
Peptic ulcer	94	66	15	13	30%

Source: C.L.H. Majoor, 1942 (16).

albumin level was less frequent and similar to the frequency found in ulcerative colitis. As it was rather difficult, if not impossible, to distinct Crohn's disease, involving the colon, from ulcerative colitis in those years, I cannot estimate with any certainty the contribution of Crohn patients to the group of 15, mentioned in the table.

Hypoalbuminemia in heart failure was frequently discussed in those days. Payne and Peters, in 1932, were among the first to establish its occurrence. Malnutrition was considered by these authors to be a distinctly more important cause of the low albumin level than hydremia, albuminuria or increased capillary permeability. In 1942 it was not possible to add supplementary evidence for alternative explanations for the cause of hypoalbuminemia in patients with a failing heart. Since 1961 however, it is known that gastrointestinal protein loss may be found in cardiac disease and may explain the low albumin level in some of these patients (Davidson et al. (18)). The relatively high frequency of low serum albumin in patients with peptic ulcer was in most cases caused by recurrent hemorrhage and in some due to infection or shock after operation.

In the first years of World War II, famine edema has not yet been a problem in Amsterdam. In Paris, however, Gounelle and his colleagues have studied 61 patients from a mental hospital in 1941 (19, 20). They found a fair correlation between serum albumin level and the extent of edema.

In severe cases serum albumin concentration was usually lower than 30 g/l. However, 6 edema patients were seen with quite normal albumin levels between 45 and 58 g/l. As no details about the technique of albumin separation were given, it is difficult to interpret these results.

In 1942 and 1943 (21, 22) Govaerts and Lequime presented interesting facts in their studies in 48 cases of famine edema seen in Brussels. Total protein levels (measured refractometrically) were slightly to definitely low in 32 of 40 patients, but the colloid osmotic pressure was reduced in all, ranging from 12 to 35 cm of H_2O. That a low metabolic rate was found in 30 of 39 patients, is not surprising on account of experiences during World War I. Pulse rates ranged from 36–84 per min. In half of the patients a definite bradycardia of less than 52 beats per min was found. It seems important to note that Govaerts et al., with Moritz and Tabora's intravenous technique, established a normal and not a too low venous pressure in 29 patients, and a too high value, ranging from 13–20 cm of H_2O, in eleven. Circulation time (sodium dehydrocholate) was prolonged in 44 of 48 patients, ranging from 18 to even 34 sec. A similar finding of circulation times ($MgSO_4$) was found in Dutch famine patients with edema by Lopes Cardozo et al. two years later (23, 24). Serum albumin, determined according to the method described by Howe (6), ranged from 31–44 g/l in these Dutch patients, that is to say distinctly above Peters' edema level of 30 g/l. The measurement of cardiac output (acetylene method) in 10 of their patients by Govaerts and Lequime is another interesting aspect of their work. Results were very low in all patients, ranging from 1.0–2.7 l/min (normal range: 3–4.3 l/min). I feel that cardiac output measurements deserve to be reinvestigated with modern techniques in severely emaciated patients (e.g. anorexia nervosa), before and after well controlled salt loads. A last series of interesting data presented by Govaerts et al. concerns arteriovenous oxygen differences in 10 of their patients. These differences were definitely increased as compared to normal values. The authors concluded that in famine edema, apart from the reduction of the osmotic pressure, a circulatory deterioration (fléchissement circulatoire) occurs that "is more important than was admitted before". In the pathogenesis of this type of edema both factors may co-operate.

In Holland, during the famine winter of 1944–1945, the official supply of food rations was limited to only 500 calories with less than 20 g of protein per day. Less than one third of this protein was from animal sources. Furthermore gas and electricity were unavailable, precluding not only

regular cooking but also almost all laboratory work. This latter circum-
stance has undoubtedly been one of the reasons why clinical investigations
on famine edema have scarcely been set up in this period. However van
Oven in Leiden (25) was able to study serum protein contents in 21 edema
patients with Gorter's modification of Langmuir's spreading technique
(26). Normal values with this method are almost identical with those of
Howe's method. Urinary chloride output was only studied in one patient,
and while in a period of massive diuresis during bed rest, so that we are
not able to derive any distinct conclusion on salt intake and output during
the Dutch famine period from van Oven's work. He stated, however, that
during this period, salt too was scantily furnished, so that it seems to be
unlikely that the mean salt intake in Holland, early in 1945, was as high as
in Munich during World War I (3). With regard to van Oven's results (Fig.
6): Although total serum protein and albumin were low in all patients with
edema during the period of starvation, albumin was only once lower than
3.0 g/100 ml. After the liberation of Holland, serum albumin became
rapidly normal in almost all patients, but edema frequently persisted and
disappeared some weeks later.

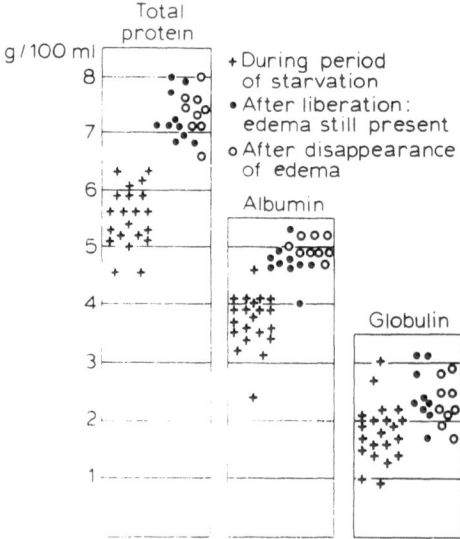

Fig. 6. Total protein, albumin and globulin concentration in sera from patients with famine
edema, studied in Leiden from April to September 1945.
(Adapted from: C van Oven (1946) (25) with permission from the author.)

During the famine period the protein content of edema fluid was found by van Oven between 0.15 and 0.40 g/100 ml, with one exception. However, in 6 patients with persistent edema for a few weeks after the liberation, a distinctly higher level of protein was found, ranging from 0.6–1.0 g/100 ml.

Shortly after the second World War, Keys and his collaborators have started a controlled experiment to study human starvation and its consequences. "From many volunteers under Civilian Public Service, 36 conscientious objectors were selected." These men subsisted on a European type of famine diet for six months. "They were to be housed and fed in the Laboratory and kept on a standardized regimen of work and general mode of life" (27, 28). In Table 3, some of the most intriguing results of this "Minnesota Semi-starvation Experiment," as Keys has called it, are compiled. The diet provided about 50 g of protein and 1760 calories. After the famine period an average of 24% of body weight was lost. Pitting edema appeared within two months, but was slight to moderate in most of the men. The decline in total plasma protein was about 10%. The 10% increase in plasma volume and the 20% reduction in hematocrit suggest that total blood volume was decreased during the edematous phase. This is consistent with the finding of low venous pressures.

The relatively constant thiocyanate space (29) has brought Keys and his collaborators to the often cited conclusion that the edema in simple caloric starvation is largely a reflection of a reduction in cellular mass.

Table 3. Compilation of results of "Minnesota semi-starvation experiment," 1944–1945 (36 volunteers on European type of famine diet for six months)

Diet	: about 50 g of protein, 1760 calories
Protein from animal origin	: about 29 g
Mean loss of body weight	: 16 kg (69.5 → 53.5 kg = 24%)
Real tissue loss	: close to 23 kg per man
Clinical edema 1 + to 3 +	: 30 of 34 men
Mean decline in plasma protein concentration	: 7.3 g/l (10%)
Decline in plasma albumin	: slight (classical Tiselius electrophoresis, only 6 samples investigated)
Venous pressure	: markedly reduced (mean 4.8 cm H_2O normal 9.7–10.3 cm H_2O)
Mean plasma volume	: from 3.13 l → 3.4 l = slight increase
Mean hematocrit	: from 46.3% → 36.6% = definite anemia
Mean thiocyanate space	: from 17.13 l → 17.88 l = almost constant, despite weight loss

Source: Ancel Keys et al., 1946 (27, 28)

This statement, to a certain degree, corroborates the large losses of tissue protein found by Weech et al. (13) in protein starved dogs. That famine edema is not simply a result of hypoproteinemia, had already been stated by earlier investigators, especially Govaerts (21, 22). Keys felt that the fall in tissue pressure can only be a minor contributing factor to edema formation. Certainly, anemia has raised the severity of edema in his subjects, in accordance with Peters' statement from 1933.

Finally Keys stated in 1947 (30) that during the three months of controlled "relief" feeding, signs of relative cardiac insufficiency appeared, with a rise of venous pressure exceeding the normal control value. Even frank congestive failure developed in one of his subjects. So in the "Minnesota Experiment" too, the "deterioration of the circulation," as it was emphasized by Govaerts et al., can be recognized.

The use of a protein free diet, providing a relatively large amount of carbohydrate and fat, for acutely uremic patients, as suggested by Borst in 1946 (31), was certainly an important development in the field of protein metabolism in clinical medicine. He presented evidence that patients in the end stage of renal disease could do well with a diet containing only 25 g of protein per day, provided that an adequate calorie intake was allowed. The serum albumin level of these patients on such diet, during months, remained normal and body weight could rise. This clinical finding again has illustrated that a sufficient calorie supply is more important to maintain nitrogen balance than a relatively large quantity of dietary protein.

One of the difficulties in interpreting older data on serum albumin in disease states is the specificity of the measurement, which was at least restricted. In American literature, Howe's method was almost exclusively used. Because the Na_2SO_4 concentration (21.5 g/100 ml), as suggested by Howe (6) for separation of albumin from globulins, was chosen on account of solubility characteristics of serum proteins, established only in 6 samples of sera derived from calves, Borst, in 1939, suggested to repeat Howe's work, in sera of healthy humans. Fig. 7 shows one of our solubility curves (16, 32). Sera from 6 volunteers were mixed and proteins were precipitated with Na_2SO_4, in concentration from 10 to almost 40 g/100 ml of serum-salt-mixtures. The nitrogen content of the filtrate was calculated as protein content in g/l of serum. The complete duplicate measurement (● ● and broken lines at the bottom of the graph) was repeated after 6 days (○ ○ and solid lines). The first conclusion from these and many other similar curves was, that precipitation with Na_2SO_4 leads to adequately reproduc-

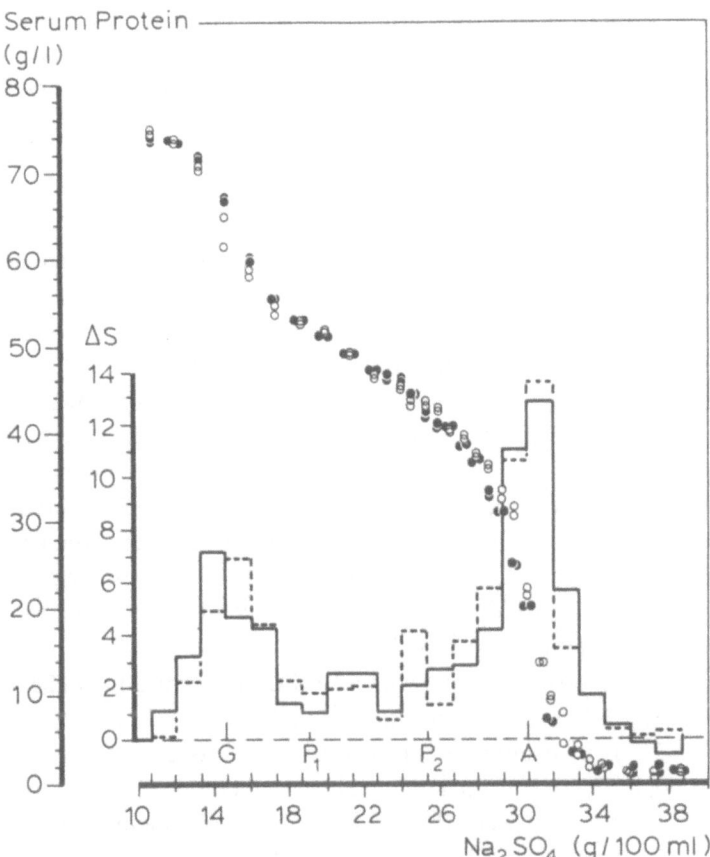

Fig. 7. Solubility curves of human serum proteins in Na_2SO_4 concentrations ranging from 10–40 g Na_2SO_4/100 ml. A mixed serum from 6 healthy individuals was studied twice with an interval of 6 days (●● and ○○). ΔS = the amount of protein precipitated by each increment of salt concentration (Δc = 1.33 g of Na_2SO_4/100 ml). The diagram at the bottom of the figure was obtained by connecting these ΔS values with broken (first experiment) and solid (second experiment) lines. For the interpretation of these datas see text.
(Adapted from CLH Majoor (1942 and 1946) (16, 32) with permission from the editor.)

ible results. A second conclusion was that in the concentration region of about 21.5 g/100 ml Na_2SO_4, no horizontal part in the solubility curve exists, as Howe had suggested. However, it is evident that steep parts in the curves do present at Na_2SO_4-concentrations of about 30.5 and 14.8 g/100 ml.

Both solubility curves were differentiated as to the quantity of protein (ΔS) precipitated with constant increments of Na_2SO_4-concentrations

(Δc = 1.33 g of Na_2SO_4/100 ml). Each ΔS was plotted at the bottom of the figure. By connecting these data with broken (first experiment) and solid (second experiment) lines, a diagram could be generated, very similar to curves obtained by the (by then recently developed) classical electrophoresis technique (33). From this similarity and complementary evidence, obtained from the literature, it was concluded that serum albumin in man starts to precipitate at a Na_2SO_4-concentration of approximately 26 g/100 ml. Maximal precipitation occurs at about 30 g/100 ml. The high peak as shown in the differentiation diagram to the right of point P_2, is caused by this fenomenon. Gammaglobulin was supposed to cause the lower peak, left of point P_1 and the protein precipitated between P_1 and P_2 was considered to be mainly other globulins. These interpretations meant that an albumin level, measured according to the method as described by Howe, is approximately 8–10 g/l higher than the real albumin content, and that the albumin fraction according to Howe contains an appreciable amount of globulins. The comparison of albumin levels derived from solubility curves, with those obtained from classical electrophoresis experiments, in highly pathological human sera, has subsequently shown (34) that both methods yielded almost identical results.

When precipitating albumin with a Na_2SO_4-concentration of 25.5 g/100 ml, Borst (35) has found a mean serum albumin level of 38.6 g/l (range 33.5–49.7 g/l) in healthy young men (n = 23) as compared to 48.0 g/l (range 42.4–57.1) if estimated by Howe's method. For healthy young women, these values were 39.3 g/l (range 34.1–45.7) and 49.6 g/l (range 45.5–54.9 g/l) respectively (n = 18). In patients with severe infections, not absolutely confined to bed and using moderate amounts of salt, edema could be expected if the serum albumin concentration, determined by the technique, using the 25.5 g/100 ml Na_2SO_4-concentration, was lower than 18 g/l.

Since 1949, paper electrophoresis has replaced salt precipation in the clinical evaluation of serum proteins almost everywhere. In our laboratory electrophoresis is performed on cellulose acetate and no corrections are made for the relatively high color affinity of albumin. The mean albumin concentration in healthy people, ascertained in this way, has been found to be 50.7 $\pm$ 3.1 g/l (n = 40, Lamers 1976 (36)). These findings are in striking accordance with the values found by Borst with Howe's original method.

Recently, Hafkenscheid and Balvert have introduced in our laboratory the method of Doumas et al. (37) to measure serum albumin with bromcresolgreen. In healthy people (n = 149) they have established a mean serum albumin content of 43 g/l (range 35.2–50.8 g/l, unpublished data). This value is similar to that found by Borst with the 25.5% Na_2SO_4 precipitation. These findings suggest that both, last mentioned, methods are adequate to come close to the true serum albumin level.

A last and certainly important development that I would like to discuss shortly, is the finding of enteric protein loss as a cause of severe hypoalbuminemia. In the literature before 1950, case histories of patients with so called idiopathic hypoproteinemia were scarce. Albright, in 1949 (38), was the first to suggest, that the disorder in albumin metabolism in these patients might not be a result of a decreased rate of synthesis, as most authors had believed before, but due to an increased rate of albumin degradation. Maimon et al, in 1947 have stated that in patients with giant hypertrophic gastritis, "unusual plasma loss from the abnormal gastric surface" (p. 420) might be the cause of the hypoproteinemia, that was found in 2 of 6 patients (39). Citrin et al. (1957, (40)) were the first to establish the occurrence of gastric protein loss in this disease.

Then in 1961 Davidson et al. (18) demonstrated enteric protein loss in patients with heart failure. One of the goals of van Tongeren's investigation (41, 42, 43) in this field was to collect information about the significance and frequency of such losses for the explanation of the hypoalbuminemia that so frequently occurs in severe heart failure.

A survey of this work is shown in Table 4 (44). In the last column of this table cases from the literature are collected up till 1969. Constrictive pericarditis proved to be the most frequent etiology of enteric protein loss in cardiac patients. Chronic rheumatic heart disease with tricuspid regurgitation, ranks certainly second. However, van Tongeren has observed two patients with this valvular lesion without enteric protein losses. Finally attention may be drawn to two patients with chronic cor pulmonale and two with emphysema without heart failure, who presented with hypoalbuminemia and definite enteric protein losses. Anoxia might well have been a factor in the pathogenesis of enteric protein loss in these two patients with emphysema without heart failure.

I realize that I have been very incomplete in this historical review of serum albumin in clinical practice. Perhaps I may conclude by forwarding some simple conclusions that have emanated from my study:

1. The colloid osmotic pressure of plasma – mainly exerted by albumin – is really an important, but not the sole, factor regulating "the absorption of fluids from the connective tissue spaces" and the pathogenesis of edema; even in patients with pure undernutrition.

Table 4. Gastrointestinal protein loss in patients with different causes of heart failure

Diagnosis	Patients in this study			Case histories collected from literature
	Within normal limits	Borderline	Definite	
1. Constrictive pericarditis	0	0	1	17
2. Pericardial effusion (L.E.D.)	0	0	0	1
3. Rheumatic heart disease with tricuspid regurgitation	2	1	2	3
4. Myocardial disease of unknown etiology	1	1	1	3
5. Chronic cor pulmonale	0	0	2	0
6. Carcinoid syndrome	0	0	0	3
7. Atrial septal defect	0	0	0	1
8. Pulmonary stenosis	0	0	0	1
9. Chronic nephritis, overhydration	0	0	1	0
10. Coronary heart disease with severe failure	3	3	0	0
Total	6	5	7	29
Emphysema without heart failure	0	0	2	0

Source: Majoor and van Tongeren, 1973 (44).

2. Abundant salt intake can convert a situation of "edema tendency" without edema (as in anorexia nervosa, carcinomatous cachexia and perhaps childhood marasmus) in overt edema.

3. In famine periods a sufficient intake of protein cannot ensure the nitrogen balance when the total caloric intake is insufficient.

4. Other factors that promote edema formation in undernutrition and probably in severe infections, are anemia, as has been stressed by Peters et al. in 1933, and probably Govaerts' "circulatory deterioration" (1942, 1943). Diminished tissue pressure and low capillary oxygen pressure may serve as significant tertiary factors.

REFERENCES

1. Starling EH: On the absorption of fluids from the connective tissue spaces. J Physiol 19:312–326, 1895–1896.

2. Epstein AA: Concerning the causation of edema in chronic parenchymatous nephritis: Method for its alleviation. Am J Med Sci 154:638–647, 1917. Reprinted in Am J Med 13:556–561, 1952.
3. Jansen WH: Die Ödemkrankheit, Studien über die Physiologie der Unterernährung und über die Ödempathogenese. Deutsch Arch Klin Med 131:144–200, 330–377, 1920.
4. Cahill GF Jr: Starvation in man. New Engl J Med 282:668–675, 1970.
5. Gamble JL: Chemical anatomy, physiology and pathology of extracellular fluid: A lecture syllabus. Fifth edition. Cambridge Harvard University Press, Chart 47, 1947.
6. Howe PE: The use of sodium sulfate as the globulin precipitant in the determination of proteins in blood. J Biol Chem 49:93–108, 1921.
7. Howe PE: The determination of proteins in blood. A micromethod. J Biol Chem 49: 109–114, 1921.
8. Govaerts P: Influence de la teneur du serum en albumines et en globulines sur la pression osmotique des protéines et sur la formation des oedèmes. Bull Ac Roy Méd Belg 7:356–373, 1927.
9. Peters JP, Eisenman AJ: The serum proteins in diseases not primarily affecting the cardiovascular system or kidneys. Am J Med Sci 186:808–833, 1933.
10. Peters JP: Body water. The exchange of fluids in man. Springfield, Baltimore, Charles C Thomas, 1935.
11. Landis EM: Micro-injection studies of capillary permeability III. The effect of lack of oxygen on the permeability of the capillary wall to fluid and to the plasma proteins. Am J Physiol 83:528–542, 1928.
12. Landis EM: The passage of fluid through the capillary wall. Harvey Lectures 32:70–91, 1936–1937.
13. Weech AA, Wollstein M, Goettsch E: Nutritional edema in the dog. V Development of deficits in erythrocytes and hemoglobin on a diet deficient in protein. J Clin Invest 16: 719–731, 1937.
14. Darrow DC, Buckman TE: The volume of the blood. II The volume of the blood and concentration of crystalloids and electrolytes in dehydration and edema. Am J Dis Child 36:248–267, 1928.
15. Chang HC: Plasma protein and blood volume. Proc Soc Exper Biol and Med 29:829–832, 1932.
16. Majoor CLH: On the significance of serum albumin determinations for the evaluation and treatment of patients with internal and surgical diseases. Thesis Amsterdam, Scheltema and Holkema, 1942. (In Dutch.)
17. Payne SA, Peters JP: The plasma proteins in relation to blood hydration. VIII. Serum proteins in heart disease. J Clin Invest 11:103–112, 1932.
18. Davidson JD, Waldman TA, Goodman DS et al: Protein-losing gastroenteropathy in congestive heart failure. Lancet 1:899–902, 1961.
19. Gounelle H, Bachet M, Sassier R et al: Sur des cas groupés d'oedèmes de dénutrition. Étude étiologique, clinique et biologique. Ration alimentaire. Bull Mém Soc Méd Hôp Paris 57:635–643, 1941.
20. Gounelle H, Bachet M, Marche J: La protidémie au cours de 6 cas d'oedèmes de dénutrition. Presse Méd 50:403, 1942.
21. Govaerts P, Lequime J: Considérations sur la pathogénie des oedèmes de famine. Bull Ac Roy Méd Belg VIe Serie, Tome VII: 260–297, 1942.
22. Govaerts P, Lequime J: Pathogénie des oedèmes de carence. Presse Méd 51:386–387, 1943.
23. Lopes Cardozo E, Eggink P: Circulatiestoornis bij hongeroedeem. Ned Tijdschr Geneesk 90:258–261, 1946.
24. Lopes Cardozo E, Eggink P: Circulation failure in hungeredema. Canad Med Ass J 54:145–147, 1946.

25. Oven C van: Protein content of blood and edema fluid in famine edema. Thesis Leiden, Eduard Ijdo, Leiden, 1946. (In Dutch.)
26. Gorter E, Blokker PC: Determination of serum albumin and globulin by means of spreading. Proc Kon Ned Acad Wetensch (Section of Sciences) 45:151–154, 1942.
27. Keys A: Human starvation and its consequences. J Am Diet Assoc 22:582–587, 1946.
28. Keys A, Taylor HL, Mickelsen O et al: Famine edema and the mechanism of its formation. Science 103:669–670, 1946.
29. Henschel A, Mickelsen O, Taylor HL et al: Plasma volume and thiocyanate space in famine edema and recovery. Am J Physiol 150:170–180, 1947.
30. Keys A, Henschel A, Taylor HL: The size and function of the human heart at rest in semi-starvation and subsequent rehabilitation. Am J Physiol 150:153–169, 1947.
31. Borst JGG: Protein katobolism in uraemia; effects of proteinfree diet, infections, and blood transfusions. Lancet 1:824–828, 1948. Reprinted in: Neth J Med 16:41–46, 1973.
32. Majoor CLH: The possibility of detecting individual proteins in blood serum by differentiation of solubility curves in concentrated sodium sulfate solutions. Yale J Biol Med 18:419–441, 1946.
33. Tiselius AA: A new apparatus for electrophoretic analysis of colloidal mixtures. Trans Faraday Soc 33:524–531, 1937.
34. Majoor CLH: The possibility of detecting individual proteins in blood serum by differentiation of solubility curves in concentrated sodium sulfate solutions. II. Comparison of solubility curves with results of electrophoresis experiments. J Biol Chem 169:583–594, 1947.
35. Borst JGG: Hongeroedeem twee en een half jaar na de bevrijding. Ned Tijdschr Geneesk 93:1036–1044, 1949.
36. Lamers CBHW: Some aspects of the Zollinger-Ellison syndrome and serum gastrin. Thesis Nijmegen, Krips Repro, Meppel, 1976.
37. Doumas BT, Watson WA, Biggs HG: Albumin standards and the measurement of serum albumin with bromcresol green. Clin Chim Acta 31:87–96, 1971.
38. Albright F, Bartter FC, Forbes AP: The fate of human serum albumin administered intravenously to a patient with idiopathic hypoalbuminemia and hypoglobulinemia. Trans Ass Am Physic 62:204–213, 1949.
39. Maimon SN, Bartlett JP, Humphreys EM et al: Giant hypertrophic gastritis. Gastroenterology 8:397–428, 1947.
40. Citrin Y, Sterling K, Halsted JA: The mechanism of hypoproteinemia associated with giant hypertrophy of the gastric mucosa. New Engl J Med 257:906–912, 1957.
41. Tongeren JHM van: Enteric protein loss. Its measurement with Cr[51] labeled plasma proteins. Thesis Nijmegen, Thoben Offset, 1967. (In Dutch.)
42. Tongeren JHM van, Majoor CLH, Kamphuys ThM: Demonstration of protein-losing gastroenteropathy. The disappearance rate of ^{51}Cr from plasma and the binding of ^{51}Cr to different serum proteins. Clin Chim Acta 14:31–41, 1966.
43. Tongeren JHM van, Reichert WJ, Kamphuys ThM: Demonstration of protein-losing gastroenteropathy. The quantitative estimation of gastrointestinal protein loss, using ^{51}Cr labeled plasma proteins. Clin Chim Acta 14:42–48, 1966.
44. Majoor CLH, Tongeren JHM van: The contribution of hypoproteinemia, due to gastrointestinal protein loss, to the formation of oedeme in patients with cardiac failure. Die Heilkunst, Sonderheft 86:15–18, 1973.

8. Causes of hypoalbuminemia

J.H.M. van Tongeren, O.J.J. Cluysenaer,
C.B.H. Lamers, P.H.M. de Mulder, and
S.H. Yap

Quantitative changes in serum albumin concentration represent an important indicator of the presence of disease or its progression or improvement. The significance of serum albumin estimations is limited to varying degrees of hypoalbuminemia, since, with the exception of cases of acute dehydration, hyperalbuminemia does not occur.

The serum albumin level depends on the balance between synthesis, catabolism (i.e. endogenous degradation and external loss) and distribution between the intra- and extravascular pool, any of which can singly or in combination be altered in disease. In clinical medicine, hypoalbuminemia is generally not the result of a single mechanism. In alcoholic cirrhosis, for example, the toxic effect of alcohol, malnutrition, hormonal changes, and the volume disturbances associated with ascites all can act together to produce hypoalbuminemia.

Serum from a healthy ambulatory adult contains about 35 to 55 g of albumin per liter, dependent on the procedure of estimation. On recumbency hemodilution lowers the serum albumin (and other proteins) by about 5 g per liter. Serum protein concentration rises during the daytime. During sleep at night it becomes lower. The range of diurnal variation of total serum protein is 10–13 g/l. The concentration of most fractions shows the same variation as the total protein level with the passage of time. As a result the relative percentage of the fractions remains the same, which fact suggests that diurnal variation is related to hemodilution and hemoconcentration.

In measuring serum albumin concentration great variation may be obtained, depending on the method being used. Four types of procedures are currently applied for the estimation of serum albumin: 1) assay of albumin by the biuret or Kjeldahl techniques after removal of globulins by salt precipitation; 2) measurement of albumin directly, by virtue of the tendency of albumin to bind certain dyes, such as bromcresol green; 3) electrophoresis followed by staining of the protein fractions; 4) assay by immunochemical procedures. The results of different techniques and also the results of different laboratories using the same method vary in general. For that reason each laboratoiy has to determine its own range of normal values.

Hypoalbuminemia is generally a reflection of a decrease in the body's total albumin pool. Such a decrease can be produced by one or a combination of three mechanisms:

1. reduced synthesis,
2. increased degradation,
2. excessive loss.

FACTORS WHICH REDUCE ALBUMIN SYNTHESIS

These include:

malnutrition
maldigestion and/or malabsorption
severe diffuse liver disease

Malnutrition

Yap et al. (1) estimated the rate of albumin synthesis (after administration of ^{14}C labelled carbonate (2)) and of the serum levels of amino acids in three patients suffering from anorexia nervosa.

For the two patients with hypoalbuminemia (serum albumin 28 and 34 g/l resp.; controls 44–55 g/l) the rate of albumin synthesis was decreased (4.9 and 9.1 g/175 cm/24 hrs. respectively; controls 22 ± SD 7). Albumin synthesis was normal (21.7) for the third patient (serum albumin 45 g/l). The serum levels of valine, isoleucine and tryptophan also were decreased in these two patients. Intravenous administration of tryptophan alone failed to increase the serum albumin level in one patient. In the other patient, a 3-week period of infusion of all essential amino acids except tryptophan failed to correct the rate of albumin synthesis or the serum albumin level. The serum albumin level rose from 37 to 47 g/l after the infusion of the essential amino acids plus tryptophan. This observation demonstrates that a reduced supply of amino acids is an important factor in the decrease of albumin synthesis and that tryptophan plays a prominent role in the regulation of albumin synthesis. Clinically as well as experimentally, amino acid mixtures can be substituted for protein in supporting albumin synthesis. This effect depends, however, upon the quality as well as the quantity of the amino acids. Tryptophan-deficient mixtures lead to deficient albumin synthesis in rats (3). The role played by tryptophan does not relate simply to the supply of this amino acid that is necessary for incorporation into albumin, since albumin contains only one tryptophan molecule. Current evidence suggests that tryptophan plays a role in ribosome-mRNA-endoplasmic reticulum stability or complexing (4).

Maldigestion and/or malabsorption

A diminished rate of albumin synthesis may be expected in patients with coeliac disease. Synthesis, however, was found to be normal in 5 of 6 untreated coeliacs (5, 6). Decreased albumin synthesis was observed in one patient (Table 1), in whom the serum concentration of the essential amino acids tryptophan was markedly and of threonine, valine, leucine and phenylalanine moderately decreased (5, 6). This patient also suffered from bacterial overgrowth in the small bowel. An excessive enteric protein loss is in general the most important factor responsible for the hypoalbuminemia in these patients (Table 1).

Samuel et al. (7) determined a decreased rate of albumin synthesis in 4 patients with tropical sprue. After parenteral nutrition with L-amino acids a remarkable improvement was observed in the rate of albumin synthesis and serum albumin concentration.

Hypoalbuminemia in patients with bacterial overgrowth in the small

Table 1. Albumin synthesis and enteric protein loss in 6 patients with coeliac sprue

age (yr)	serum albumin (g/l)	enteric protein loss (ml plasma/day)	albumin synthesis (g/175 cm/day)
62	34	110	7
32	25	360	27
44	33	215	20
52	44	80	29
50	27	330	23
60	18	400	21
controls (n = 15)	44–55	< 30	22 ± 7

bowel is not rare. Some of these patients demonstrate an intestinal protein loss, which is not always high enough to explain the hypoalbuminemia. In these latter cases the hypoalbuminemia may be due to a decreased synthesis of albumin as the result of an insufficient delivery of amino acids to the liver due to malabsorption (as a result of mucosal injury to bacteria) or to bacterial degradation of amino acids in the small bowel. It is well known, that bacterial growth in the upper small bowel can disturb normal digestion and absorption of nutrients. Hence steatorrhea and a decreased vitamin B12 absorption are often observed in these patients (8). Bacterial overgrowth. in the small bowel has been recognized in 11 patients (9). In all but one patient hypoalbuminemia, from 22 to 43 g/l, was observed. The rate of albumin synthesis was markedly decreased in 3 patients (7.0 to 10.5 g/175 cm/24 hrs.). The concentration of the essential amino acids tryptophan, valine, isoleucine, leucine and phenylalanine was abnormal low in these 3 patients compared to the remaining 8 patients. Jones et al. (10) observed a reduced rate of albumin synthesis in a patient with bacterial overgrowth. The concentrations of most of the essential amino acids were decreased in this patient, while after treatment with antibiotics the amino acid levels and the albumin synthesis were normalised.

Severe diffuse liver disease

Impaired hepatic function is a cause of depressed serum albumin levels. The liver has a considerable reserve potential. Only 10 to 25% of the hepatic cells appear to be essential to provide a normal level of albumin synthesis. Since liver damage must be severe for serum albumin levels to be reduced (11), situations that affect all liver cells, such as toxins or massive hepatic necrosis (hepatitis), are much more effective in producing hypoalbuminemia than diseases such as cirrhosis, which leave a number of hepatic cells unaffected (12). The most important toxin from the clinical point of view is alcohol, which has been shown to cause disruption of the endoplasmic reticulum of the hepatocyte of man (13) and to result in decreased albumin synthesis in perfused animal livers (14). The secretion of albumin is also highly sensitive to the membrane damage produced by such toxins as carbon tetrachloride. Of 6 female patients with chronic hepatitis or liver cirrhosis (serum albumin range 20 to 43 g/l) the rate of albumin synthesis was normal in 3, increased in 1 and obviously reduced in 2 patients. (Table 2) (6). These 2 patients progressed into hepatic coma and died respectively several weeks and a few months after the investigation.

Table 2. Albumin synthesis in patients with diffuse liver disease

Age (yr)	Diagnosis	Ascites	Serum albumin (g/l)	Total bilir. (μmol/l)	GOT (U/l)	GPT (U/l)	Albumin synthesis (g/175 cm/day)
59	chron. act. hepatitis	–	43	6	22	24	16
56	cirrhosis	+	29	52	28	10	7
54	alcohol. hepatitis	+	20	281	90	13	6
44	alcohol. hepatitis	--	38	10	22	24	44
47	cirrhosis	–	39	47	19	16	19
30	cirrhosis	+	22	6	6	4	21
controls (n = 15)			44–55	< 15	< 15	< 15	22 ± 7

INCREASED ALBUMIN DEGRADATION

To indicate the importance of an increased degradation for the development of hypoalbuminemia, some data on serum albumin and albumin synthesis in 3 patients with bacterial diseases are shown in Table 3 (6). The rate of albumin synthesis was not very depressed. The serum concentrations of amino acids were normal. An increased albumin degradation seems, therefore, the most important factor in such situation. The same results were observed in 2 of 3 patients suffering from chronic rheumatoid arthritis (serum albumin 36, 37 and 47 g/l; albumin synthesis 34, 20 and 17 g/175 cm/24 h), in a patient with deep vein thrombosis of the leg and pulmonary embolism (serum albumin 31 g/l; albumin synthesis 13 g/175 cm/24 h) and in a patient with hyperthyroidism (serum albumin 35 g/l; albumin synthesis 19 g/175 cm/24 h) (6).

EXCESSIVE ALBUMIN LOSS

A well known and important factor, which causes hypoalbuminemia is an excessive protein loss.

A classical example is the *nephrotic syndrome*, characterised by massive proteinuria, hypoproteinemia, edema and lipidemia. This clinical syndrome has a number of causes, including glomerular diseases, metabolic

Table 3. Serum albumin and albumin synthesis in patients with bacterial diseases

Age (yr)	Diagnosis	Serum albumin (g/l)	Albumin synthesis (g/175 cm/day)
69	pyelitis	29	15
57	periappendicular abscess	29	15
23	endocarditis lenta	26	14
controls			
(n = 15)		44–55	22 ± 7

diseases, collagen vascular disease, circulatory disturbances or toxins. A small amount of protein is normally present in the glomerular filtrate. This is reabsorbed by the tubular cells. In the process of reabsorption a proportion of the protein undergoes catabolism. It is thought that this is one of the reasons why in heavy proteinuria the body is at a dual disadvantage in that protein is not only lost in the urine but that there is an increased fractional catabolic rate due to increased protein reabsorption by the nephron. The urinary loss of protein initiates a reduction in the size of the total exchangeable albumin pool. The absolute degradation rate of albumin decreases in conjunction with this decrease in pool size, but the fractional degradation rate for albumin is increased. Albumin synthesis may be decreased, normal, or slightly increased, in fact only one-third to one-half of nephrotic patients have albumin synthesis rates that are elevated above normal (15).

Protein loss from the skin can occur in conditions such as extensive burns, allergic reactions, psoriasis and toxic "epidermal necrolysis". The changes that occur in albumin metabolism in patients with severe burns represent the complex interaction of a number of factors. Most important is the loss of albumin from and into the burned area. A considerable increase in capillary permeability in association with the burn results in a significant loss of albumin from the intra-vascular into the extravascular space. An amount of albumin equivalent to one plasma pool may be lost from the body, and an equivalent amount may be sequestered in the extravascular space during the first four days following a burn in patients with involvement of 50%, or more of the body surface (16). Another drawback is the fact that lymphatics are assumed to be unable to return extravascular albumin back to the plasma because lymphatics and lymphnodes are overloaded by material derived from the burn area (17). Loss of skin may also result in the loss of a significant amount of the exchangeable albumin pool because of the fact that skin contains a major portion of the extravascular albumin (18). Albumin synthesis may be decreased or increased.

Enteric protein loss is a frequent cause of hypoalbuminemia. The loss of albumin is part of a bulk protein loss, which is not related to the molecular weight of the protein. Excessive gastrointestinal albumin loss, in association with the loss of other serum proteins, has been demonstrated in conjunction with a number of gastrointestinal disorders of diverse causes (Table 4) (20–23). It has been shown that from 2 to 60 percent of the intravascular pool may be cleared into the gastrointestinal tract each day (20). In some patients with excessive enteric protein loss gastrointestinal symptoms are absent and edema may be the only clinical manifestation. For this reason, protein-losing gastroenteropathy should be suspected in all patients with unexplained hypoalbuminemia. When albumin is lost into the gastrointestinal tract, it is catabolised rapidly into its constituent amino acids, which are subsequently absorbed. These amino acids are transported to the liver by the portal circulation and are available for the resynthesis of albumin. Hypoalbuminemia develops when the rate of albumin degradation exceeds the liver's capacity to synthesize albumin (21). Protein-losing gastroenteropathy may result in some degree of increase in albumin synthesis (4) and is generally characterized by an increase in the fractional and absolute degradation rates of albumin (20). Other factors play a role too, e.g. the influence of mucosal disease of the intestine on the absorption and bacterial degradation of proteins and amino acids.

Hypoalbuminemia is an important clue to the presence, progression or improvement of gastrointestinal disorders. This point has to be stressed, because serum albumin estimations are extremely helpful in detecting gastrointestinal disease. To measure gastrointestinal protein loss the use of proteins labelled with ^{51}Cr is recommended and protein loss into the gastro-

Table 4. Some disorders associated with protein losing gastroenteropathy

---

Inflammations of the G.I. tract (gastritis, Crohn's disease, colitis)
Tumours of the G.I. tract (carcinoma, lymphoma)
Celiac sprue
Bacterial overgrowth of the small bowel
Radiation enteropathy
Disturbance of intestinal lymph flow
   – congenital lymphatic abnormalities
    (intestinal lymphangiectasia)
   – inflmmation or tumour infiltration in mesenteric lymphnodes
   – lymph congestion in thoracic duct (right heart failure, constrictive pericarditis)

---

intestinal tract can be expressed in terms of a clearance rate of ^{51}Cr labelled proteins (23–25).

Hypertrophic gastritis, characterized by considerable hypertrophy of the gastric mucosal folds, is often associated with hypoalbuminemia and in severe cases with the presence of edema. The cause of the disease is unknown. Clinically, patients present with upper abdominal pain, edema and melena, but symptoms may be absent. In a series of 13 cases (m/f: 7/6; age 34–84) we found hypoalbuminemia in all but one case (Fig. 1). Five patients visited their physician only because of edema of the legs, 2 presented with melena and 8 with epigastric pain, heartburn and belching. There was a good correlation between serum albumin concentration and enteric protein loss (Fig. 1).

Crohn's disease is a well-known chronic inflammatory disease of the small intestine and colon and associated with hypoalbuminemia in a very high percentage. In a series of 170 cases from our department 89% of the patients had hypoalbuminemia at their first visit (Fig. 2). Of 116 estimations of enteric protein loss performed on 87 patients, 92% proved abnormal (Fig. 3). Patients with a normal enteric protein loss were usually examined because of diarrhoea after an ileocoecal resection to exclude a recurrence. There was a significant negative correlation between enteric protein loss and serum albumin. The correlation with total serum protein was less pro-

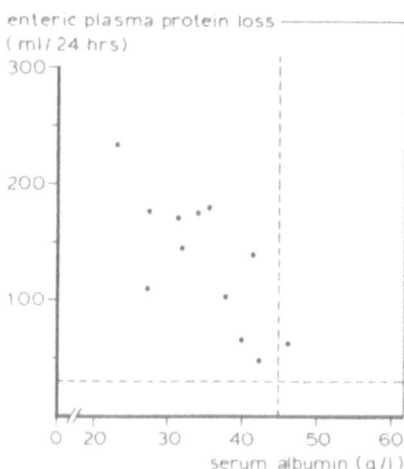

Fig. 1. Relationship between enteric protein loss and serum albumin in 12 patients with hypertrophic gastritis.

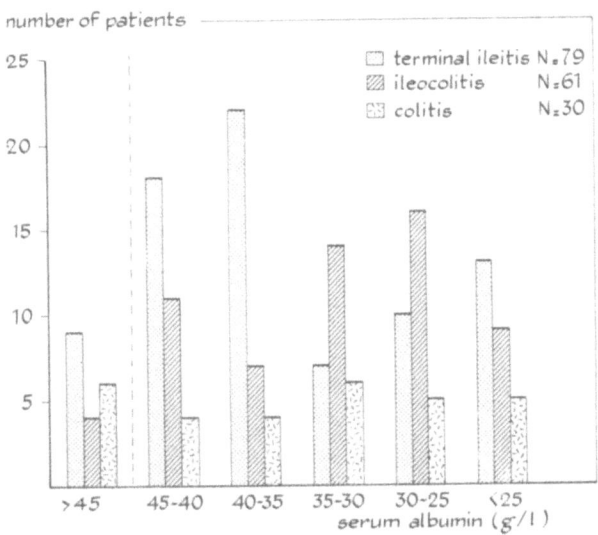

Fig. 2. Serum albumin level in 170 patients with Crohn's disease of the small and/or large bowel at the time of their first visit to the outpatient department. (Reproduced from van Tongeren and Eekhout; with permission of the authors and publisher).

nounced (Fig. 4) and absent with γ-globulin. A reduction of total serum protein was only present in 60% of the patients, so determination of total serum protein is a less reliable way to trace patients with inflammatory bowel disease than serum albumin estimation. This is because in these patients a fall in serum albumin is often accompanied by a rise in serum globulins. The total serum protein therefore remains within normal limits unless the enteric protein loss is extensive (26).

Hypoalbuminemia is also very common in patients with coeliac sprue. Cluysenaer and van Tongeren (5) diagnosed hypoalbuminemia in 83% of 36 untreated patients (Fig. 5). Coeliac sprue is also associated with enteric protein loss in almost every case (Fig. 6 and Table 1). During treatment with a gluten-free diet serum albumin became normal after 2 to 8 months (Fig. 7).

Peptic ulcer disease is sometimes a manifestation of the Zollinger-Ellison (ZE) syndrome. This syndrome is characterized by signs and symptoms of peptic ulcer, diarrhea, acid hypersecretion and gastrin producing tumours. To distinguish patients with simple peptic ulcer disease from patients with ZE-syndrome an easily performed laboratory

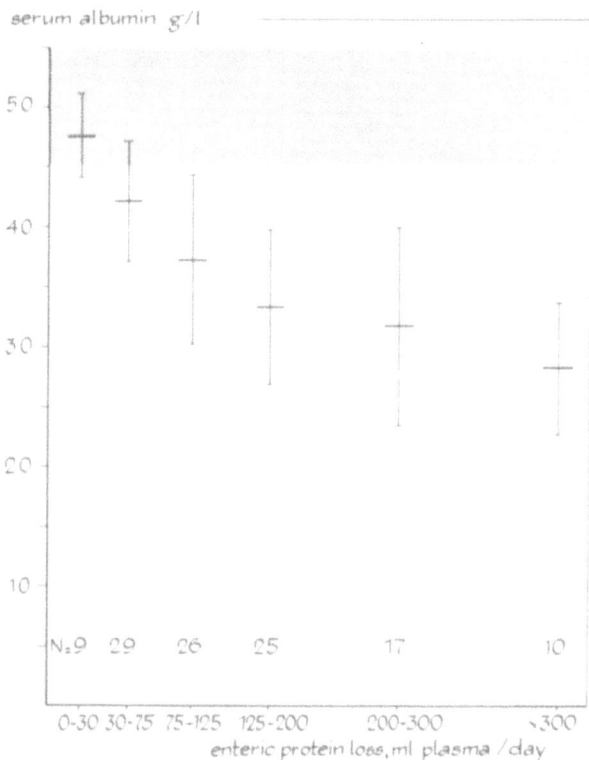

Fig. 3. Relationship between enteric protein loss and serum albumin level: 116 estimations in 87 patients with Crohn's disease, divided into 6 groups according to extent of enteric protein loss. The mean values of serum albumin ±1 SD are marked. The shaded area represents the normal range of serum albumin (reproduced from van Tongeren and Eekhout (26); with permission of the authors and publisher).

test would be of great help as a first screening procedure. Serum albumin estimation appears to be such a test (27). Patients with just a duodenal or stomal ulcer had normal or borderline serum albumin levels, whereas 15 of 20 patients with ZE-syndrome had hypoalbuminemia (Fig. 8). Total gastrectomy induced a rise in serum albumin in all 8 patients, who underwent such a procedure. In 7 serum albumin became normal, but in one of these patients with metastatic gastrinoma the serum albumin concentration remained reduced. In 4 patients total gastrointestinal protein loss was measured and in 3 protein loss from the stomach (Table 5). The intestine was the main site of protein loss in 2 cases. Loss from the stomach wall was

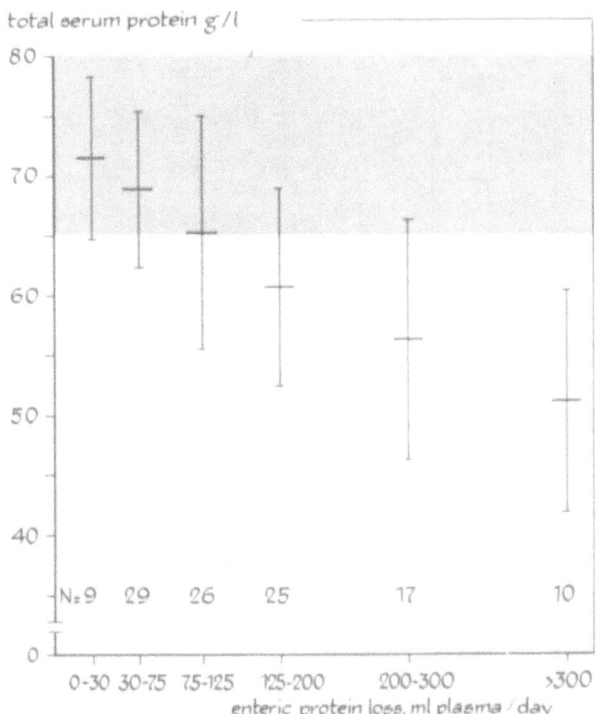

Fig. 4. Relationship between enteric protein loss and total serum protein: 116 estimations in 87 patients with Crohn's disease divided into 6 groups according to extent of enteric protein loss. The mean values of total serum protein ±1 SD are marked. The shaded area represents the normal range of total serum protein (reproduced from van Tongeren and Eekhout; with permission of the authors and publisher).

only moderately increased. Damage to the jejunal mucosa resulting from the low pH in the proximal small bowel is the major cause of the high enteric protein loss in these patients.

Obstruction of intestinal lymph flow can be another cause of excessive enteric loss of plasma proteins. This obstruction may be due to disorders of intestinal lymphatics (primary intestinal lymphangiectasia), to an inflammatory process or neoplasms involving mesenteric lymphatics and lymph nodes (retroperitoneal fibrosis, Whipple's disease, regional enteritis, lymphomas, mesenteric sarcomas etc.) or to an increased intestinal lymphatic pressure (constrictive pericarditis, tricuspid regurgitation, primary myocardial disease). These disorders may be associated with dilatation of the mucosal and mesenteric lymphatics of the small intestine.

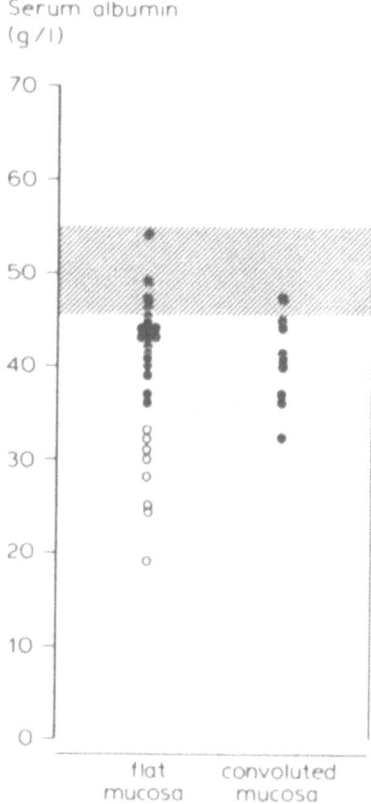

Fig. 5. Serum albumin in untreated celiac sprue. The serum levels are drawn separately for patients with a flat and with a convoluted jejunal mucosa. Statistical analysis revealed no significant difference between both groups. Hollow dots represent patients with peripheral edema, and solid dots those without edema. The shaded area represents the range of normal values (reproduced from Cluysenaer and van Tongeren (5); with permission of the authors and the publisher).

Obstruction of intestinal lymphatics often, but not always, results in loss of lymphocytes into the lumen, along with the plasma losses. The finding of lymphocytopenia is helpful in narrowing the cause of protein loss to those conditions which lead to lymphatic stasis. Primary intestinal lymphangiectasia is a disorder in which there is protein loss associated with dilatation of the mucosal and mesenteric lymphatics of the small intestine. It is but one component of a diffuse congenital hypoplasia of the lymphatics. Most cases are first recognized in children; in more severe

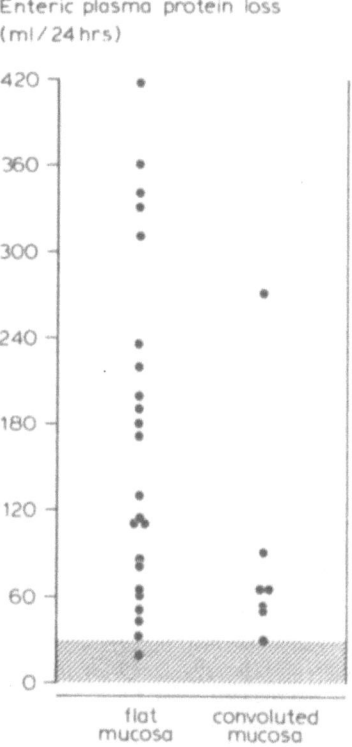

Fig. 6. Enteric plasma protein loss in 30 untreated patients with celiac sprue. The results are drawn separately for patients with a flat and with a convoluted jejunal mucosa. The shaded area represents the range of normal values (reproduced from Cluysenaer and van Tongeren (5); with permission of the authors and the publisher).

cases, manifestations are already present at birth or shortly thereafter. Peripheral edema is a prominent feature of the condition because of the lymphatic abnormalities that are generally present in the lower extremities as well as the hypoproteinemia that occurs secondarily to the intestinal protein loss. Other clinical features seen in this condition include lymphocytopenia, hypocalcemia, reduced serum immunoglobulin levels, weight loss and weakness, partially due to hypovolemia.

Congestive heart failure may be associated with some degree of hypoalbuminemia. This fact was already mentioned in 1932 by Payne and Peters (28). This decrease in serum albumin is due to hemodilution. In 1961 Davidson et al. (29) detected considerable gastrointestinal protein loss as an important cause of hypoproteinemia in 4 patients with con-

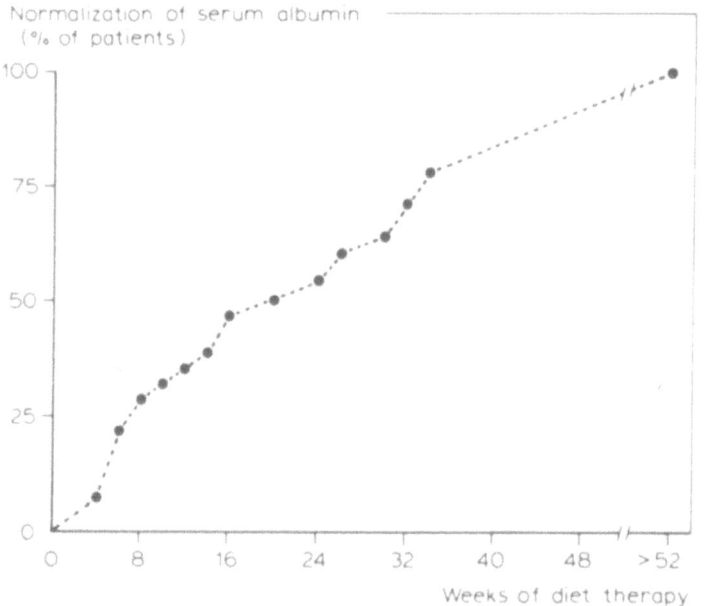

Fig. 7. Serum albumin and gluten-free diet. Both the extent and the rate of normalization of serum albumin levels on diet therapy in all 28 followed-up patients with hypoalbuminemia are recorded (reproduced from Cluysenaer and van Tongeren (5); with permission of the authors and the publisher).

gestive heart failure. Three of them had chronic constrictive pericarditis and the fourth a congenital atrial septal defect. Enteric protein loss has also been described in other cardiac disorders. An example of hypoalbuminemia due to constrictive pericarditis is the case history of a 35 year old housewife, who suffered from progressive edema since 17 years. In 1977 constrictive pericarditis was diagnosed. Serum proteins and enteric protein loss before and after surgical decortication were as follows:

	before	after	normal
total serum protein	35	68	65–75 g/l
serum albumin	22	46	44–55 g/l
serum γ-globulin	3	10	7–13 g/l
enteric protein loss	590	16	< 30 ml/day

What is the explanation of enteric protein loss in constrictive pericarditis? Sustained systemic venous hypertension seems to be a prerequisite, which increases lymph flow. A second condition is a functional

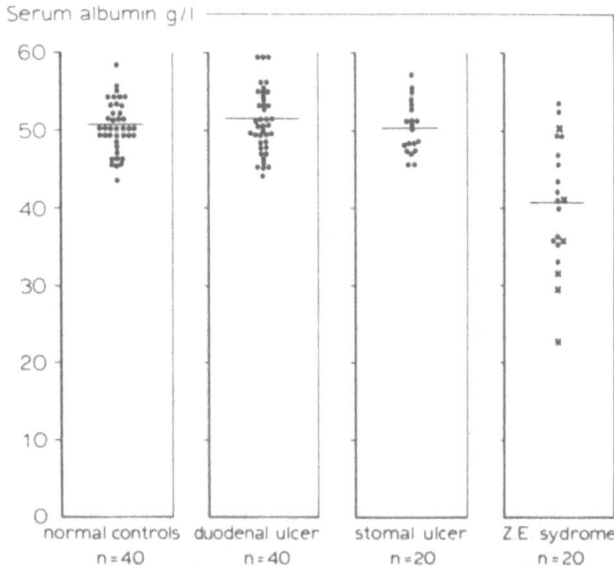

Fig. 8. Serum albumin concentration in normal subjects and patients with duodenal ulcer, stomal ulcer and Zollinger-Ellison (ZE) syndrome. x: patients with metastatic gastrinoma. (Reproduced from Lamers et al. (27); with permission of the authors and publisher).

obstruction to normal lymph drainage from the thoracic duct into the subclavian vein as the result of an excessive lymph flow. This causes a high lymphatic pressure which is transmitted to the lymph vessels of the bowel wall. Dilatation (and rupture) of these channels may occur with gastro-intestinal loss of lymphocyte-rich lymph.

The study of gastrointestinal protein loss has provided a better under-standing of the pathogenesis of the hypoproteinemia seen in association

Table 5. Enteric protein loss in 4 patients with the Zollinger-Ellison Syndrome

Age (yr)	Serum albumin (g/l)	Gastric protein loss (ml plasma/day)	Total gastrointestinal protein loss (ml plasma/day)
39	34	37	326
17	35	28	100
37	46	39	58
43	49	–	16
controls	44–55	< 12	< 30

with gastrointestinal disease and may be the only way of indicating the intestinal tract as diseased, since many patients have hypoproteinemia and edema as the only clinical manifestations of their gastrointestinal disorder.

REFERENCES

1. Yap SH, Hafkenscheid JCM, van Tongeren JHM: Important role of tryptophan on albumin synthesis in patients suffering from anorexia nervosa and hypoalbuminemia. Am J Clin Nutr 28:1356–1363, 1975.
2. Hafkenscheid JCM, Yap SH, van Tongeren JHM: Measurement of the rate of synthesis of albumin with ^{14}C-carbonate: a simplified method. Z Klin Chem 11:147–151, 1973.
3. Munro HN: Factors in regulation of liver protein synthesis. In: Plasma Protein Metabolism, MA Rothschild, TA Waldmann (eds), New York, Academic, 1970, p 157–167.
4. Rothschild MA, Oratz M, Schreiber SS: Albumin synthesis. N Engl J Med 286:784–757, 816–821, 1972.
5. Cluysenaer OJJ, van Tongeren JHM: Malabsorption in Coeliac Sprue. The Hague, Martinus Nijhoff, 1977.
6. Yap SH: De synthese en afbraak van albumine bij de mens onder normale en pathologische omstandigheden. Thesis University of Nijmegen. Meppel, Krips Repro, 1975.
7. Samuel AM, Jarnum S, Jeejeebhoy KN: Influence of parenteral L-isomeric amino acids on absolute albumin synthesis rates in tropical sprue. Scand J Gastroent 4: suppl 3, 51, 1969.
8. Neale G, Gompertz D, Schönsby H, et al: The metabolic and nutritional consequences of bacterial overgrowth in the small intestine. Am J Clin Nutr 25:1409–1417, 1972.
9. Yap SH, Hafkenscheid JCM, van Tongeren JHM, et al: Rate of synthesis of albumin in relation to serum levels of essential amino acids in patients with bacterial overgrowth in the small bowel. Europ J Clin Invest 4:279–284, 1974.
10. Jones EA, Craigie A, Tavill AS, et al: Protein metabolism in the intestinal stagnant loop syndrome. Gut 9:466–469, 1968.
11. Rothschild MA, Oratz M, Zimmon D, et al: Albumin synthesis in cirrhotic subjects with ascites studied with carbonate-^{14}C. J Clin Invest 48:344–350, 1969.
12. Peters T, Jr: Serum albumin. Adv in Clin Chem 3:37–111, 1970.
13. Rubin E, Lieber CS: Alcohol-induced hepatic injury in non-alcoholic volunteers. N Engl J Med 278:869–876, 1968.
14. Rothschild MA, Oratz M, Mongelli J, et al: Alcohol-induced depression of albumin synthesis: Reversal by tryptophan. J Clin Invest 50:1812–1818, 1971.
15. Jensen H, Rossing N, Anderson SB, et al: Albumin metabolism in the nephrotic syndrome in adults. Clin Sci 33:445, 1967.
16. Birke G: Regulation of protein metabolism in burns. In: Plasma Protein Metabolism, MA Rothschild, TA Waldmann (ed), New York Academic, 1970, p. 415–425.
17. Hamback LD, Rittenbury MS: Response of the reticuloendothelial system to thermal injury. Surg Forum 16:47, 1965.
18. Katz J, Bonorris G, Sellers AL: Extravascular albumin in human tissues. Clin Sci 39:725–729, 1970.
20. Waldmann TA, Wochner RD, Strober W: The role of the gastrointestinal tract in plasma protein metabolism. Am J Med 46:275–285, 1969.

21. Waldmann TA: Protein-losing enteropathy. Gastroenterology 50: 422–443, 1966.
22. Rothschild MA, Oratz M. Schreiber SS: Albumin metabolism. Gastroenterology 64:324–337, 1973.
23. Waldmann TA: Protein-losing gastroenteropathies. In: Gastroenterology, vol 2, third edition, HL Bockus (ed), Philadelphia, Saunders Comp, 1976, p 361–385.
24. Tongeren JHM van, Majoor CLH, Kamphuys TM: Demonstration of protein-losing gastroenteropathy. The disappearance rate of ^{51}Cr from plasma and the binding of ^{51}Cr to different serum proteins. Clin Chim Acta 14:31–41, 1966.
25. Tongeren JHM van, Reichert WJ, Kamphuys TM: The quantitative estimation of gastrointestinal protein loss, using ^{51}Cr-labelled plasma proteins. Clin Chim Acta 14:42–48, 1966.
26. Tongeren JH, Eekhout AL: Criteria to assess the severity of Crohn's disease and the effect of treatment. In: The management of Crohn's disease. IT Weterman, AS Pena, CC Booth (eds), Amsterdam, Excerpta Medica, 1976, p 153–158.
27. Lamers CBH, Hafkenscheid JCM, Yap SH, et al: Serum albumin levels in patients with the Zollinger-Ellison syndrome. Gastroenterology 73:975–979, 1977.
28. Payne SA, Peters JP: The plasma proteins in relation to blood hydration. VIII. Serum proteins in heart disease. J Clin Invest 11:103–112, 1932.
29. Davidson JD, Waldmann TA, Goodman DS, et al: Protein-losing gastroenteropathy in congestive heart failure. Lancet 1:899–902, 1961.

9. The colloid osmotic pressure in cardiac disease

J. Gerbrandy, S.J. Smith, and H.G. van Eijk

The relation between cardiac function and plasma volume and as a consequence between cardiac function and plasma proteins is contradictory (Table 1). On the one side cardiac failure causes retention of water and salt and consequently a hemodilution. As a result, the central venous pressure (CVP) rises and the total protein content and also the colloid osmotic pressure (COP) of the plasma fall. If the cardiac function is restored, the edema is excreted, a hemoconcentration occurs and the CVP falls again. On the other hand, a rise of CVP causes in itself an increase of capillary hydrostatic pressure and this, according to the Starling-mechanism would result in a hemoconcentration with a rise of plasma protein (1). Recovery of cardiac failure attended with a fall of CVP, causes a hemodilution and a fall of plasma protein.

Both processes can be demonstrated in patients with congestive heart failure. As shown in Fig. 1, digitalis is administered to a patient with congestive heart failure and gross edema. Immediately after the intravenous injection of 1.5 mg Digoxin the second mechanism can be observed: a rapid fall of CVP of about 6 cm water is accompanied by an immediate hemodilution with a slight fall of hemoglobin content. After this, a tremendous diuresis occurs together with a marked hemoconcentration as indicated by the rise of hemoglobin.

Table 1.

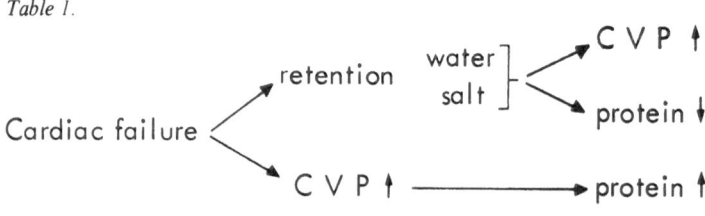

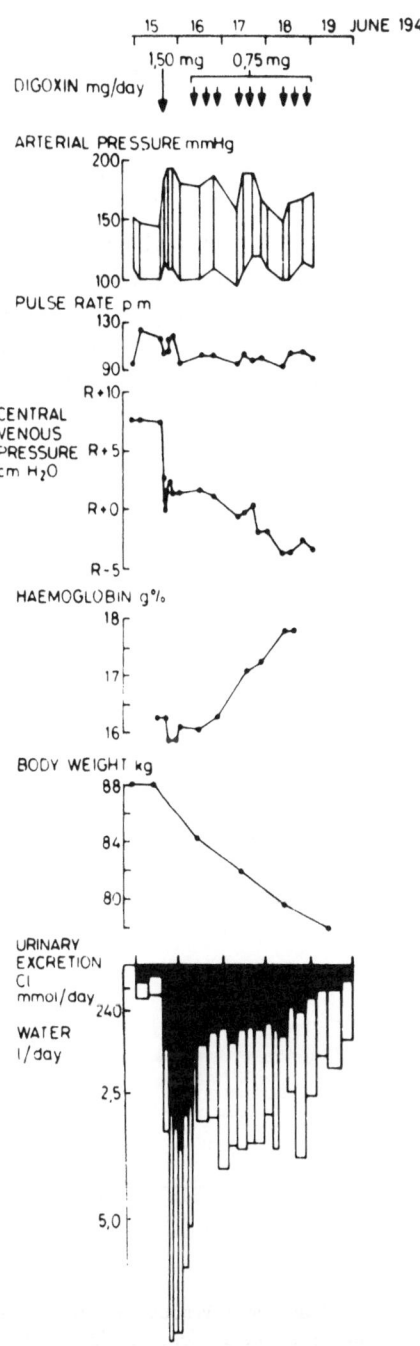

Fig. 1. Changes of CVP, hemoglobin and body-weight after intravenous injection of digoxin in a 70-year old man with heart failure and gross edema.

To emphasize the influence of CVP on plasma volume in cardiac disease, we have examined the relation between the fall in central venous pressure and the fall in hemoglobin content in 24 patients with congestive heart failure following intravenous injections of digitalis glycosides and aminophyllin. As can be seen in Fig. 2, a fall of CVP of 1 cm water correlates with a fall of hemoglobin of about 1% or with an increase of plasma volume of about 50 ml. This correlation has been demonstrated again in our recent observations in 14 patients with acute myocardial infarction (2).

Fig. 3 shows the mean results of the repeated determinations of hemoglobin and hematocrit in these 14 patients. After 3 days, a mean hemoconcentration of 2.2% occurs most probably by a rise of CVP. Afterwards

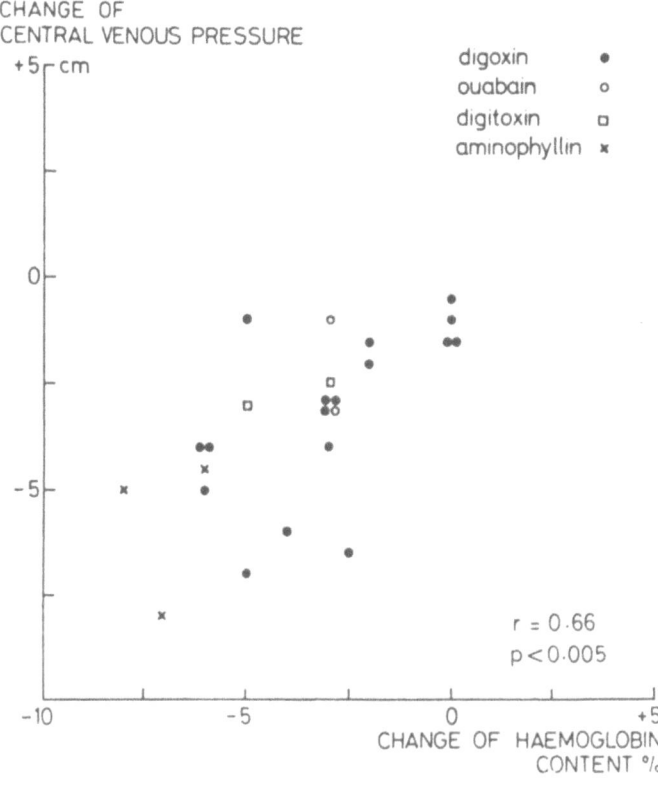

Fig. 2. Relation between the fall in central venous pressure and the fall in hemoglobin content in 24 cases of congestive heart failure following intravenous injection of digitalis glycosides and aminophylline.

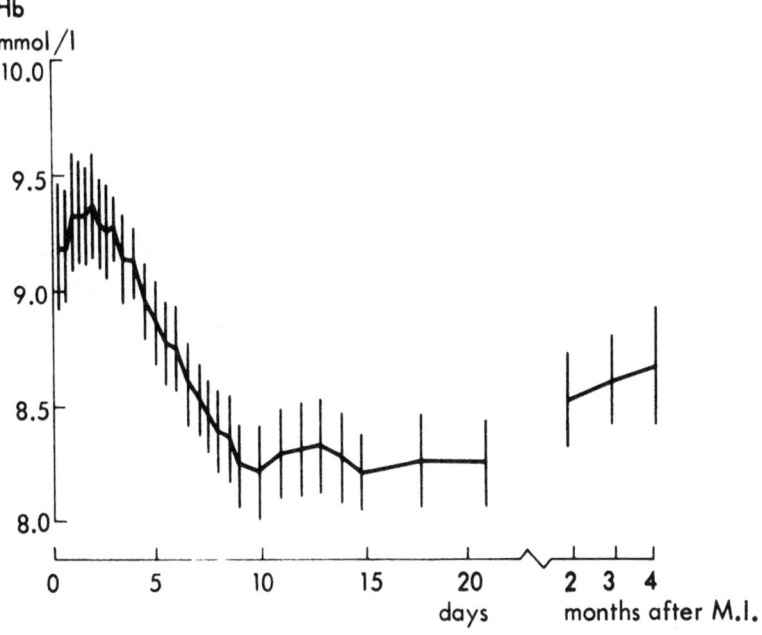

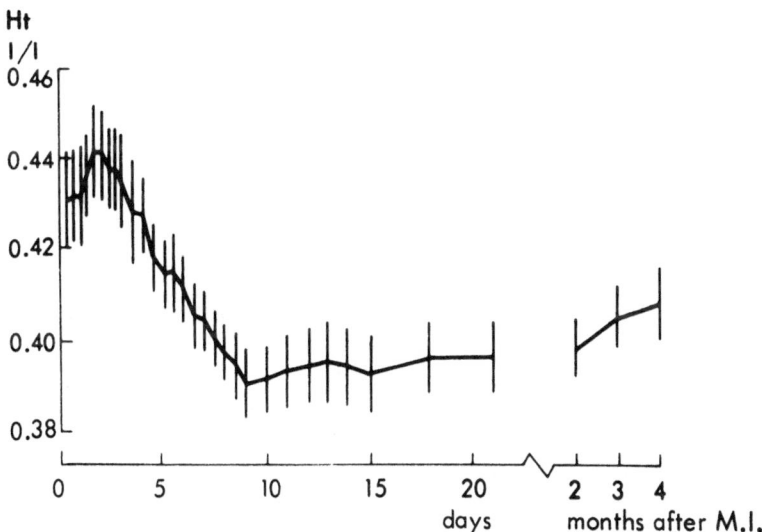

Fig. 3. The mean results of repeated determinations of hemoglobin and hematocrit in 14 patients with acute myocardial infarction.

a hemodilution is seen presumably as a result of retention of water and salt. The assumption that the initial rise of hemoglobin is caused by a rise of CVP is substantiated in Fig. 4. The 6 patients *with* lung edema – and presumably with a high CVP – show a much greater initial rise of hematocrit than the 8 patients *without* lung edema (4.5% versus 1%). Unfortunately the CVP in our patients is not followed systematically, but Buchwalsky et al. (3) have shown in their study of 25 patients with myocardial infarction that the CVP (measured intravascularly) increased in greater extend in patients with lung edema than in patients without lung edema.

However, our findings concerning the course of the colloid osmotic pressure of the plasma were not quite similar to these of hemoglobin and hematocrit. For determination of COP, see Bos et al. (4). As shown in Fig. 5 the COP of the 6 patients with lung edema rises only shortly, and in the 8 patients without lung edema a continuous fall can be seen.

The cause of this discrepancy is demonstrated in Fig. 6. During the first

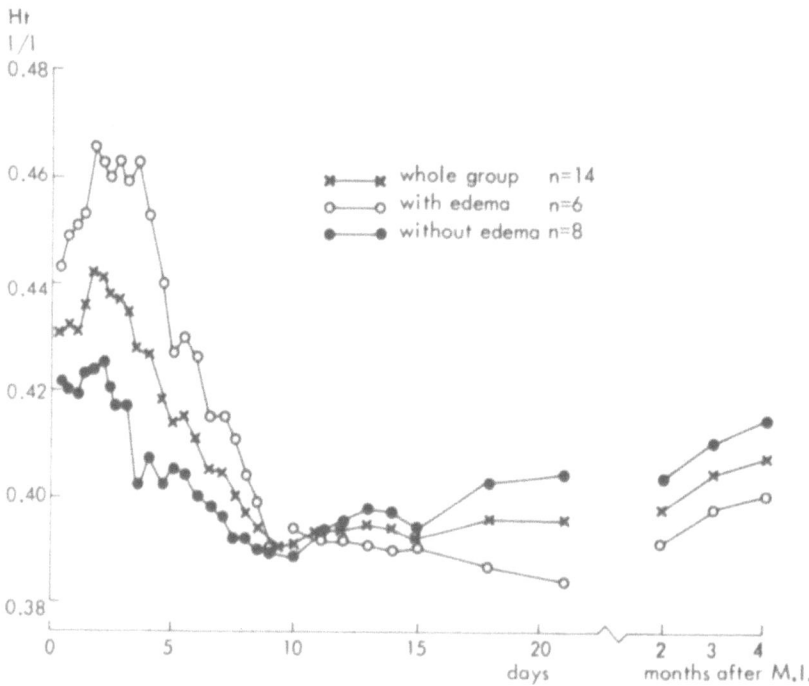

Fig. 4. The course of hematocrit in 14 patients with acute myocardial infarction, differentiated in 6 patients with and 8 patients without lung edema.

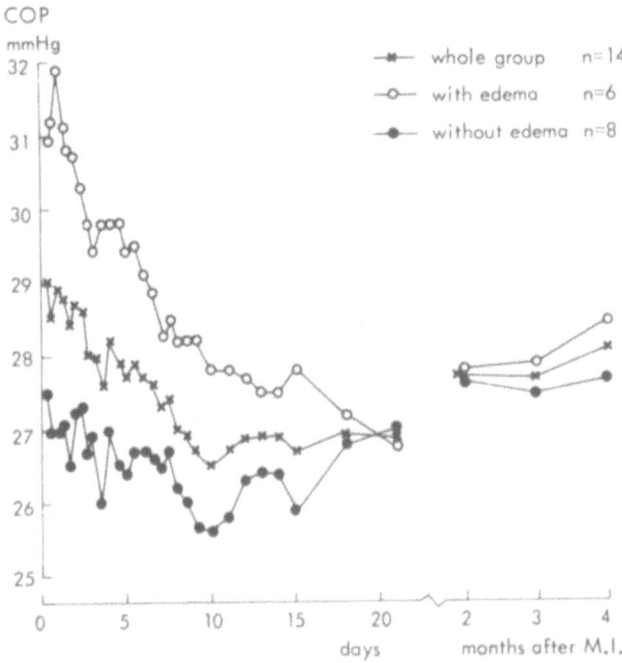

Fig. 5. The course of COP in 14 patients with acute myocardial infarction, differentiated in 6 patients with and 8 patients without lung edema.

3 days, the hematocrit and total plasma protein concentration rise initially, but the COP and plasma albumin concentration fall. It is apparent in this study that the decrease of albumin concentration is associated with the fall of COP, but the total plasma protein concentration remains unchanged after the initial rise. Therefore, we may conclude that the loss of albumin is replaced by other proteins which are unable to compensate the loss of colloid osmotic pressure of albumin.

As can be seen in Table 2 on the 10th day after infarction, a marked hemodilution is observed as indicated by the fall of hematocrit of nearly 10%. In the same period the albumin has fallen with 17.6%. However, notwithstanding this hemodilution and the marked fall of plasma albumin concentration the total plasma protein concentration remains practically the same. This may be attributed to the flow of so-called acute phase proteins into the plasma, that is to say globulins made by the liver as a reaction to tissue necrosis in the body. Between day 3 and day 10, the plasma albu-

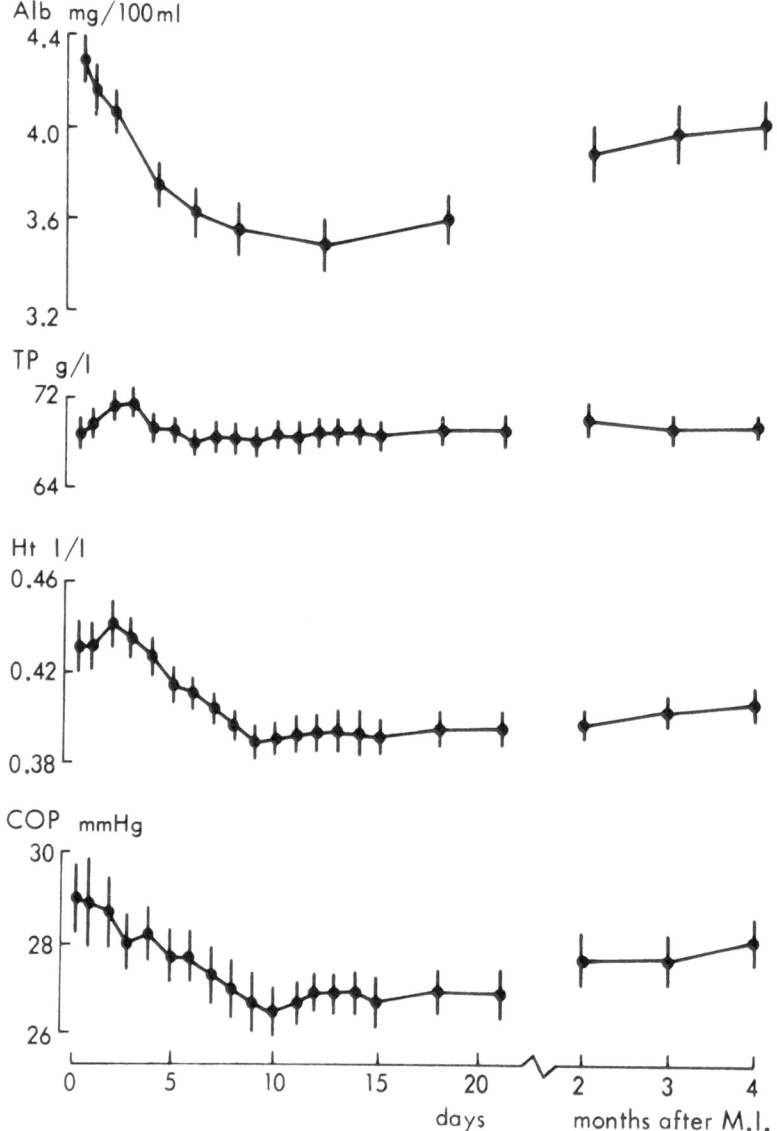

Fig. 6. The mean course of hematocrit, total protein, albumin and COP in 14 patients with acute myocardial infarction.

min concentration falls with 13.1% and the COP decreases with 7.0%. The ratio between the molecular weight of albumin and mean molecular weight of globulin is about 7:15. Therefore if the loss of albumin is replaced by the

Table 2.

14 patients with acute myocardial infarction

	after 2 days	after 9 days	after 120 days
alb	5.1 % ↓	17.6 % ↓	6.3 % ↓
Tot. Prot.	2.9 % ↑	- .6 % ↓	-.7 % ↑
Ht	2.3 % ↑	9.5 % ↓	5.3 % ↓
COP	1.0 % ↓	7.9 % ↓	2.8 % ↓

gain of globulin, the COP has to be decreased with $7/15 \times 13.1 = 6.1$. This calculation compares satisfactorily with the 7% we found.

As tissue necrosis occurs somewhere in the body, in our cases myocardial infarction, the liver is stimulated to produce acute phase globulins (Figs. 7 and 8). In our series a highly significant correlation appeared to exist between the extent of myocardial infarction, estimated as the function of production of a specific myocardial enzyme (α-hydroxybutaric acid dehydrogenase (α-HBDH) and the production of the globulins by the liver: C-reactive protein, α l-antitrypsin, α l-acid glycoprotein, haptoglobin and fibrinogen. Apart from these *positive* acute phase proteins, there are also the so-called *negative* acute phase proteins, i.e. plasma proteins which fall as a result of tissue necrosis, namely albumin and transferrin. As shown in Fig. 8, the plasma concentrations of albumin and transferrin appear to fall substantially after myocardial infarction, however, the correlation between the extent of myocardial infarction and the fall of albumin was not very close.

The main question remains: what is the meaning of this fall of albumin: 18% in 10 days. To show that the fall of plasma albumin concentration is not only a result of hemodilution, the concentration of albumin is corrected by the hematocrit according to the formula $1/1 - $ Ht. As shown in Fig. 9 a fall of corrected albumin concentration still can be observed (11.6%) at the 5th day. However, it is important to note that the hematocrit in such periods of time is not a reliable parameter. To elucidate this question we tried to define the correlation between the fall of albumin and the fall of COP. Experimentally we determined the COP's related to the actual concentrations of albumin.

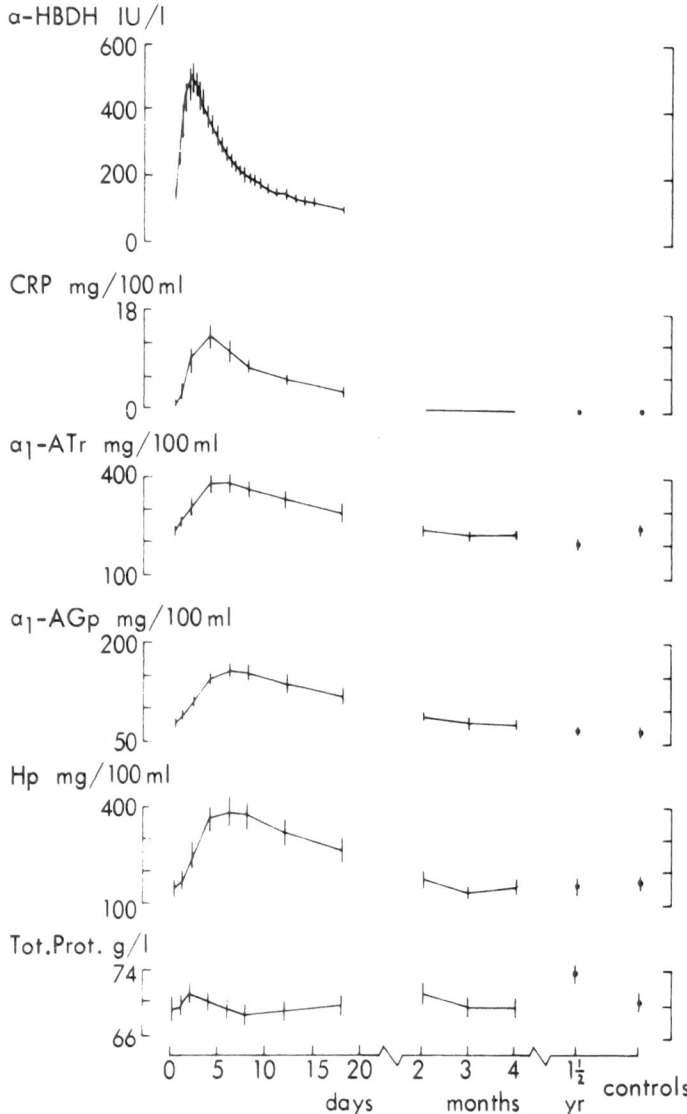

Figs. 7 and 8. The rise of the myocardial enzyme α-HBDH, the rise of the positive acute phase proteins α₁-anti-trypsin, α 1-acid glycoprotein, haptoglobin and fibrinogen; the fall

Fig. 10 shows the mean albumin – COP curve of our 14 patients. It appears that this curve deviates from the actual plasma-COP curve that we have determined before (Fig. 6). The difference of these 2 curves is explained by the increased concentrations of globulins in the plasma (the acute phase proteins).

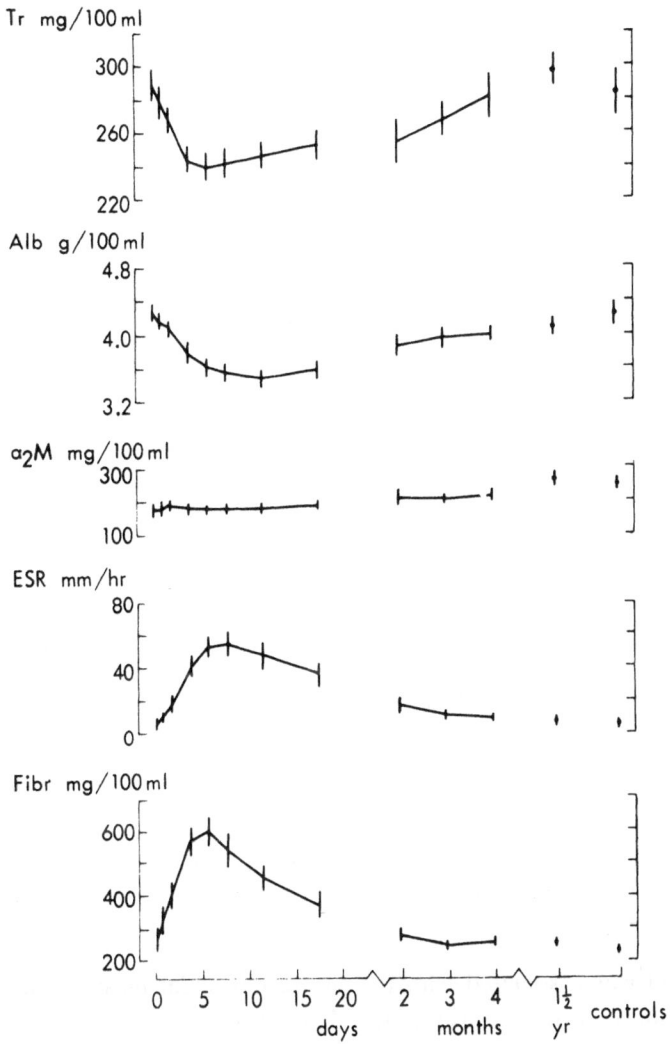

of the negative acute phase proteins transferrin and albumin and the even course of total protein and α 2-macroglobulin in 14 patients with acute myocardial infarction.

As given in Table 3 molecular masses of positive and negative acute phase proteins (5) are compared and also of $\alpha2$ macroglobulin, that is not affected by tissue necrosis and that did not change in our patients with myocardial infarction. In each patient, the fall of molecular mass of the negative acute phase proteins (albumin and transferrin, both carrier

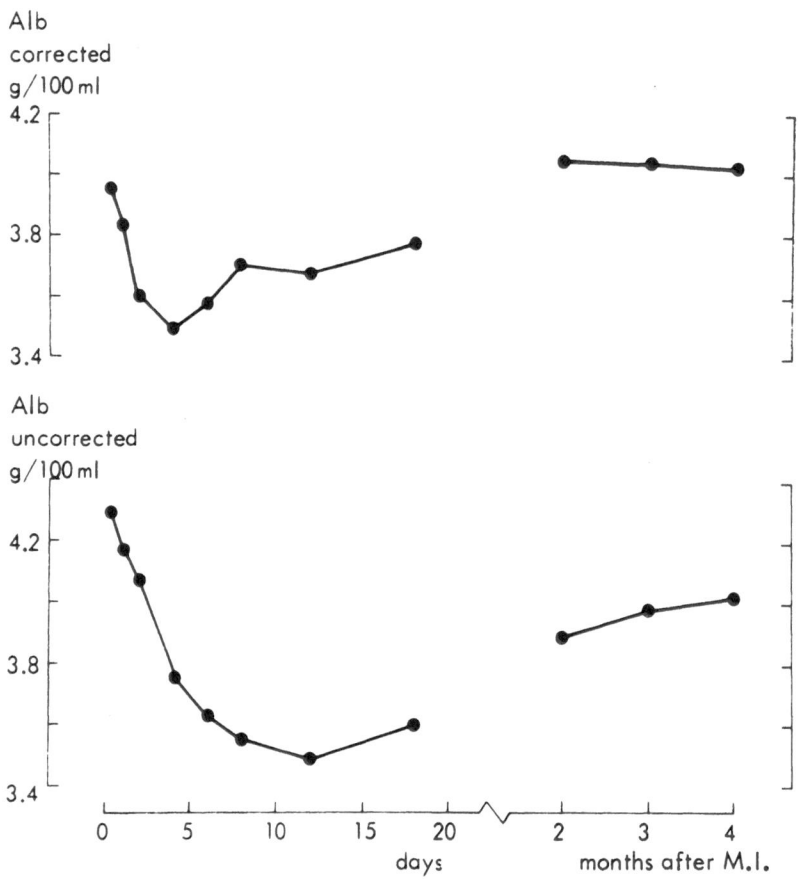

Fig. 9. The course of albumin uncorrected and albumin corrected by hematocrit in 14 patients with acute myocardial infarction.

proteins) was associated with the rise of molecular mass of the positive acute phase proteins, also called defense proteins (C-reactive protein, fibrinogen, haptoglobin, α1-acid glycoprotein and α1-antitrypsin). In 11 of 14 patients a statistically significant correlation appeared to exist (Table 4).

Then, the question arises: What is the exact mechanism of regulation? What is the determinating factor: COP, albumin, total protein or the circulation?

The COP falls, but this happens in a not stabilised condition of hemo-dilution. The albumin may have diffused into the infarction itself or into

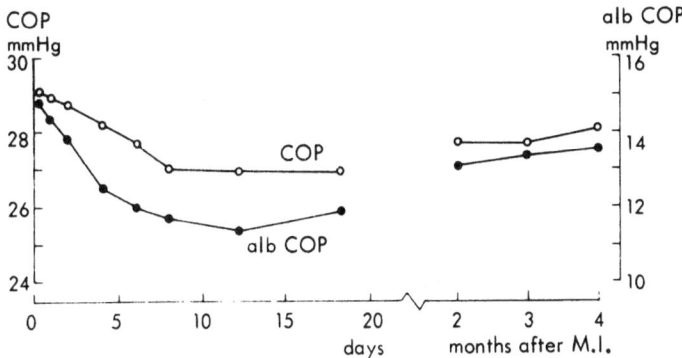

Fig. 10. The mean course of COP and/of albumin – COP of 14 patients with acute myocardial infarction.

Table 3. Molecular weight

Molecular weight

albumin	69.000
transferrin	76.000
a_2-macro-globulin	820.000
C-reactive protein	127.000
fibrinogen	341.000
haptoglobin	100.000
a_1-acid glycoprotein	44.100
a_1-anti-trypsin	45.000

the interstitial space. But on the other hand the significant correlation between the fall of negative and the rise of positive acute phase reactants suggest a regulation of plasma albumin concentration as a colloid osmotic adaptation to the acute production of globulins. Moreover, in the acute inflammatory plasma protein response, the total colloid osmotic increase of acute phase reactants, complement and immunoglobulins is approxi-

Table 4.

$$\text{Correlation} \quad \frac{\text{fall mol. neg. acute phase proteins}}{\text{rise mol. pos. acute phase proteins}}$$

11/14 patients

r 0.664 – 0.929
p <0.05 – <0.001

mately the same as the total colloid osmotic decrease of the carrier proteins (6–7).

Finally the capacity of the liver to produce proteins is perhaps limited, and a forced production of defense proteins by the liver may result at the expense of the production of albumin as major protein synthesized in the liver.

The importance of COP in the fluid movement into and from the lung capillaries is illustrated in Table 5. There is no doubt that in this special region fluid movement from capillaries into interstitial lung tissue has to be prevented and this is achieved by a comfortable excess of plasma COP above the hydrostatic pressure in the lung capillaries. In patients with acute myocardial infarction the lung capillary pressure, estimated by the pulmonary capillary wedge pressure (PCW) is known to be elevated, and lung edema threatens if the PCW amounts to 18 mm Hg. However, lung edema can sometimes occur in patients with a lower PCW and patients with a PCW higher than 18 mm Hg developed no lung edema.

Therefore, we have studied COP and PCW in 30 patients with acute myocardial infarction (Fig. 11). (8). All patients had an indwelling catheter

Table 5.

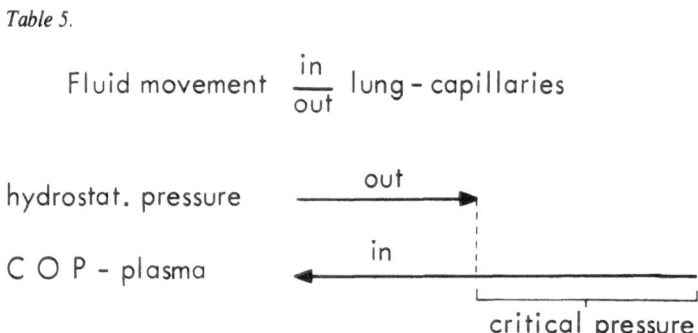

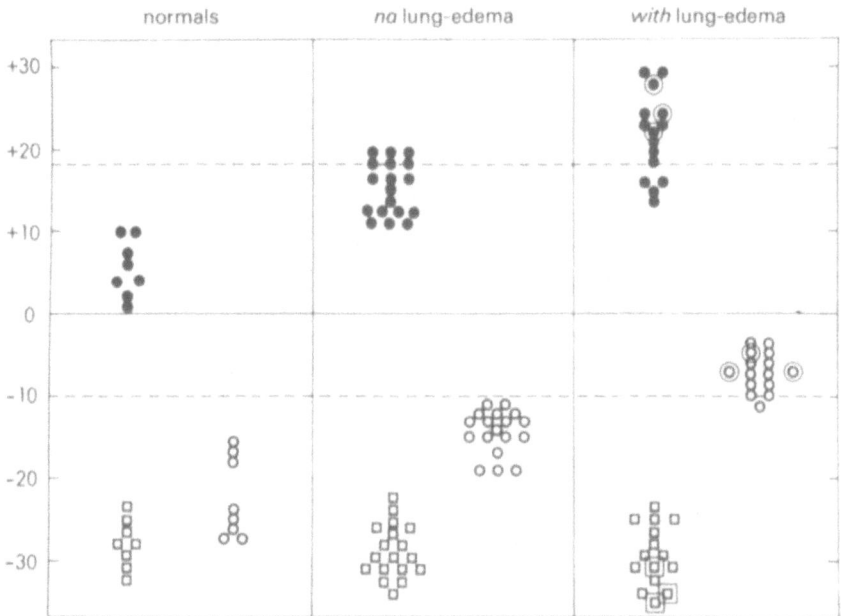

Fig. 11. Measurements of PCW (pulmonary capillary wedge pressure, black dots), of colloid osmotic pressure of the plasma (squares) and of critical pressure (open circles) in 8 normals, 18 patients with acute myocardial infarction without lung edema and 12 patients with 15 attacks of lung edema.

for repeated measurement of PCW: 10 patients developed no lung edema and in 12 patients, 15 periods of lung edema were observed. The values of PCW and COP were not significantly different between patients with and without lung edema. However, if the critical pressure was calculated, that means the difference of these two values, a clear distinction could be seen between the 2 groups at 10–11 mm Hg. It can therefore be concluded that the COP next to the PCW plays an important role in the pathogenesis of lung edema.

REFERENCES

1. Gerbrandy J, Molhuysen JA: Relation between central venous pressure and blood volume during treatment of heart failure. Neth J Med 16: 146–154, 1973.
2. Smith SJ: Plasma eiwitten en colloid osmotische druk na het acute myocardinfarct. Thesis, Rotterdam, 1977.
3. Buchwalsky R, Zeh E: Zentraler Venendruck und klinische Symptomatologie beim frischen Herzinfarct. Zeitschr für Kreislaufforsch 61:124, 1973.

4. Bos G, Smith SJ, Van Eijk HG: De colloid osmotische druk. Achtergronden en klinische betekenis. Chemie en Techniek 32:252–258, 1977.
5. Schultze HE, Heremans JF: Molecular biology of human proteins. vol I. Nature and metabolism of extracellular proteins. Elsevier-Amsterdam, 1966.
6. Laurell CB: Determination and interpretation of plasma proteins. Australian Family Physician 5, Special Issue Dec. 1976.
7. Eijk HG van: Moderne aspecten van de serum eiwitanalyse. Bepaling en interpretatie van plasma eiwitspiegels. Tijdschr Med Anal 32: 341–349, 1977.
8. Smith SJ, Hagemeijer F, Gerbrandy J, Esseveld MR: The significance of colloid osmotic pressure and pulmonary capillary wedge pressure in pulmonary edema secondary to acute myocardial infarction by man. Neth J Med 19: 118–126, 1976.

10. Changes in plasma albumin concentration and drug action

E. J. ARIËNS AND A. M. SIMONIS

INTRODUCTION

In order to discuss and understand the role of plasma albumin in drug action, it is good to consider what the function of albumin in the organism is. The appearance of *albumin* in the line of *evolution* can give an indication in this respect. It turns out that albumin becomes a predominant plasma protein in the era where animals left the oceans and became terrestrians (land animals) (see Table 1) (1). This even is manifest in the metamorphosis of the tadpole, a water animal where little or no albumin is available to the frog (1). Also in the development from fetus via neonatus to adult the plasma albumin concentration increases (2).

Table 1. Evolutionary aspects of plasma proteins and drug metabolism

Species[a]	Plasma protein %	Oxidative N-demethylation[c]	Phenol glucuronidation[d]	Species[b]
man	6.5	19 ± 2	21 ± 3	mouse
dog	6.1–6.7	15 ± 2	46 ± 13	rat
turtle	4.8	26 ± 8	85 ± 22	pigeon
crocodile	3.69	4 ± 0.6	8.9 ± 2.3	lizard
frog	1.5–4.3	1.6 ± 0.45	1.26 ± 0.47	frog
skate	2.4–3.1	1.1 ± 0.30	1.72 ± 0.25	trout
menhaden	0.72–2.9	0.71 ± 0.28	1.9 ± 0.33	goldenorfe
goosefish	1.4–2.2	0.86 ± 0.23	2.68 ± 0.65	carp

[a] (1).
[b] (5, 12).
[c] μmoles formaldehyde formed per gram fresh liver tissue/hour.
[d] μmoles p-nitrophenol glucuronidation per gram fresh liver tissue/hour.

Note the increases at the switch from water to land animals.

One of the well recognized functions of albumin in this respect is the colloid osmotic action, widely discussed and reasonably well understood both from the physiological as from the pathophysiological point of view. Besides its colloid osmotic action, essential for fluid household, albumin has other vital functions, also related to the switch from aquatic animal to terrestrian animal. As long as the animal lives in the water, it can freely exchange and thus easily dispose via its gills of water-soluble and poorly water-soluble, more lipid-soluble agents in a practically unlimited fluid compartment. This holds true both for agents of endogenous origin (for instance, bilirubin) and for agents taken up from the environment, xeno-biotics, of which the organism has to dispose because of their potential toxicity. Once on land, the disposal of relatively water-soluble agents is still possible in the limited volume of urine produced daily. This is not possible anymore for the poorly water-soluble, more lipophilic agents. Remarkably, in the line of evolution, in the era of the transition from water animal to land animal, enzyme systems evolve, e.g. the mixed-function oxidase in the liver, and conjugating enzymes, capable of converting more lipid-soluble agents into end-products which are good water-soluble, as a rule less toxic and suitable for excretion with the urine (Table 1) (3, 4, 5). The main aspects of drug elimination are summarized in Fig. 1 (6). Extremely lipid-soluble agents tend to a temporary storage in adipose tissue. If they are resistant against metabolic conversion, they are sequestrated there for a long time. DDT is an example of such an agent. Plasma albumin also serves as a carrier system for free fatty acids and thus is an important factor in fat metabolism, which is indispensable for the supply of calories especially in warm-blooded animals. Also in this respect the evolutionary development in plasma albumin makes sense. Interestingly, with the en-hancement of the pharmacon-metabolizing capacity of the liver induced by various lipophilic agents with relatively long half-life times in plasma, e.g. phenobarbital, there is a concomitant increase in the albumin synthesis (7).

Water-soluble agents tend to restrict themselves in their distribution mainly to the extracellular fluid compartment where they are readily avail-able for renal excretion, by ultrafiltration or by active excretion, while they have little tendency to tubular reabsorption or to penetration and accu-mulation in the cells; in this way, their toxicological risks are well under control. Poorly water-soluble, lipophilic agents, however, would tend to accumulate in the cells while their concentration in the extracellular water is very low. Such compounds would be hardly available to the metabolic

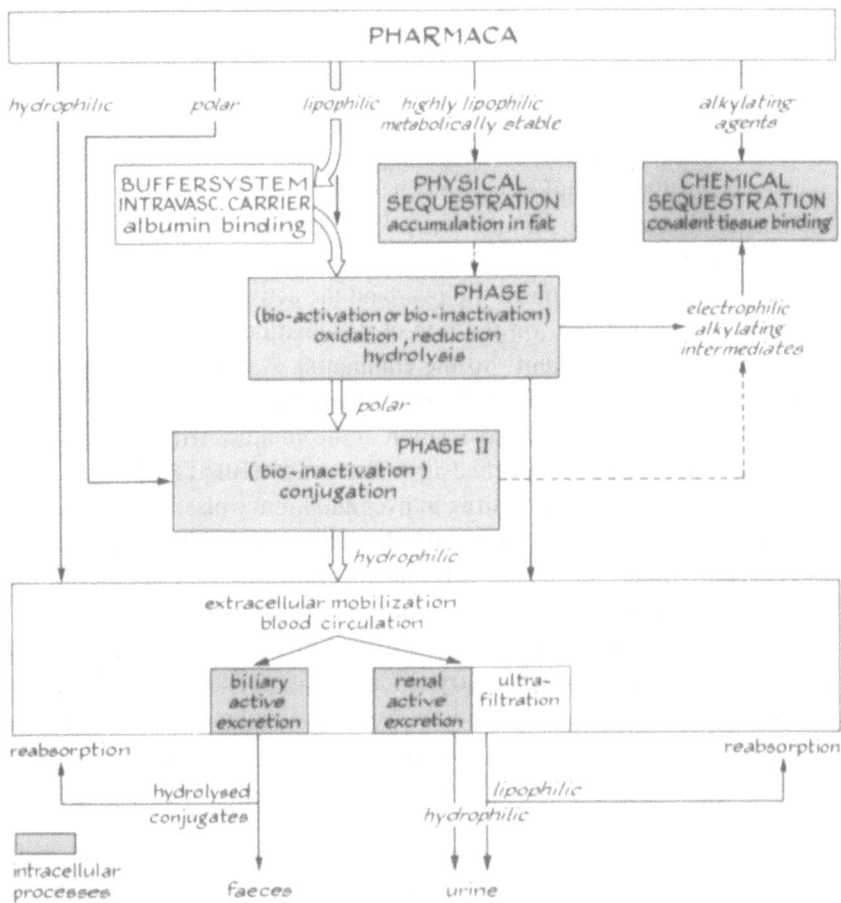

Fig. 1. Schematic representation of the main aspects of drug metabolism.

systems in the liver, generally involved in their elimination. Accumulation of such agents in the body cells and thus intoxication, may be avoided by a buffer system which relatively strongly binds the lipophilic agents. In that way the free concentration in the extracellular fluid can be kept extremely low, and the exposure of the tissue cells to such agents strongly limited. In order to make the poorly water-soluble, lipophilic agents nevertheless readily available for the liver enzyme systems involved in the elimination, a carrier system is needed to increase the load of these agents in the intravascular fluid compartment and thus to facilitate transport to the liver cells. The enzyme systems concerned are usually indicated as drug-metabolizing enzyme systems, they, however, are involved in the disposal of both body-own and body-foreign lipid-soluble agents. The evolutionary increase in the concentration of plasma albumin with a relatively high affinity for such agents constitutes the buffer capacity as well as the intravascular transport system required by land animals (8, 9). Whether the load of drug, circulating in the albumin-bound form, is available for the enzyme systems involved in biochemical conversion in the liver and the active transport systems in the kidney is dependent on the rate of dissociation of the albumin-drug complex and on the affinity to the eliminating systems. The drug metabolizing enzymes have a relatively high affinity for the lipid soluble agents. For most drugs the rate of dissociation of the complex with albumin is so high that equilibrium is reached in milliseconds (10). This implies that practically the whole load of drug in liver and kidney plasma flow is available for the eliminating systems mentioned, such that the plasma flow through the organs becomes a determinant factor for the clearance of the agents concerned. Drugs for which the rate of dissociation of the drug-albumin complex is extremely low are exceptions to this rule. Suramin, for instance, a prophylactic against trypanosomiasis, persists in the plasma for several weeks after one single dose. Some radiopaques, e.g. 3-hydroxy-2,4,6-triiodo-α-ethylhydrocinnamic acid, persists in the plasma-protein bound form for years after a single dose (11). These agents are pseudo irreversibly bound to albumin.

The reduction in the free concentration as a result of binding to albumin reduces the rate of ultrafiltration of the compounds in the glomerular capillaries – the albumin-bound form is excluded from ultrafiltration – and thus tends to delay renal excretion. Since, however, predominantly lipophilic agents – agents which after glomerular ultrafiltration are reabsorbed to a large extent in the tubuli by passive diffusion via the tubulus wall – are involved, their renal excretion also in the absence of albumin anyway would be small. Binding to albumin has no great effect on the rate of renal elimination of the lipophilic agents therefore. The predominant route of elimination for more lipophilic agents is via metabolic conversion. The more hydrophilic agents which are primarily excreted with the urine (little or no passive tubular reabsorption takes place) are not or to a minor degree bound to albumin. In fact albumin binding reduces the principally useless and for the tubular cells potentially risky circuit (the glomerulo-tubulary cycle) in which the lipophilic agents concerned would participate.

Two major adaptations have taken place in the development of aquatic to terrestrian animals:

1. the development of *liver enzyme systems* involved in the detoxification and elimination of undesirable endogenous or exogenous pollutants (3, 4, 5). The question arises whether also the *transport systems* involved in *active renal excretion* evolved simultaneously. The conjugating enzyme systems preparing the products of oxidative metabolic conversion for active renal excretion did appear simultaneously with the drug-oxidizing enzymes in the liver.
2. a strong increase in plasma albumin, serving from the one hand as a *colloid osmotic agent* essential for the fluid dynamics and fluid homeostasis (1) and from the other as a *buffer system* capable to keep away potentially toxic lipophilic agents from the tissue cells and as an effective *transport system* to channel these agents to the enzyme systems in the liver converting them to more water-soluble products suitable for rapid renal elimination. Similar adaptations take place during ontogenesis (1, 9, 12, 13). Thus plasma albumin forms part of a vital defence system against internal pollution with lipid-soluble agents, including the various drugs to which man is exposed.

Remarkably enough, along the line of evolution mankind is supplied with a defence system against the risks of internal pollution, also an aspect of modern medicine. Insufficiency of this defence system undoubtedly increases the patient's risks of drug exposure. This is a sufficient reason to discuss the relationship between plasma albumin concentration and drug action, the topic of this paper.

ALBUMIN – DRUG BINDING

Both therapeutic and adverse effects of drugs and chemical agents in general are a simple function of the plasma concentration (14, 15, 16, 17). In general, in the protein-bound form the agents cannot diffuse into the tissue cells and may be only exceptionally active in this form on the cell surface (insulin bound to a solid carrier, sepharose, appears to be still active on fat cells (18). In the free (unbound) form drugs freely exchange between plasma and interstitial fluid. An exception has to be made for a few macromolecular agents, such as plasma extenders. Penetration into the central nervous system (passage of the blood-brain barrier) and into the fetal compartment as well as into the intracellular fluid is easy for non-ionized lipid-soluble agents but difficult or impossible for highly water-soluble and polar agents such as quaternary ammonium compounds, for instance curare. Such agents usually have their sites of action, receptors, on the cell surface.

Albumin, present in plasma in a concentration of 40 g per liter, which makes 120 g in total plasma, and in the interstitial fluid in a concentration of 12.5 g per liter which makes about 150 g in total interstitial fluid, is the main protein component for drug binding in the extracellular compartment. Binding to other plasma proteins, erythrocytes and tissue components (19) will not be discussed here. Albumin binding is relatively strong for agents with a hydrophobic (lipophilic) structure which as a rule are relatively poorly soluble in water (8). Generally spoken, there are *three types of binding sites*, namely for acidic compounds, for basic compounds and for neutral compounds. On these sites *mutual displacement* by the particular types of agents, for instance displacement of acids by acids, takes place. Part of the clinically significant drug interactions resulting in adverse effects for the patient find their origin in such displacement (20, 21, 22, 23, 24).

A clear instance of the function of albumin as a buffer for potentially toxic agents is the binding of bilirubin (25). In hyperbilirubinemia, plasma albumin is to a large extent saturated with bilirubin. Displacement of bilirubin from albumin results in a shift of bilirubin, now in the unbound form, to the extravascular extracellular compartment, and thus to an enhanced exposure of the tissues; as a result thereof it penetrates into and accumulates in the cells, leading, for instance, to kernicterus (24, 26, 27) (see

Table 2. Mortality among premature infants with a prophylactic treatment with two types of antibacterial regimens (reproduced from reference 26)

Treatment	No. of infants	Mortality rate (%)	Kernicterus deaths (% autopsies)	Mean peak serum bilirubin (mg %)*
Sulfisoxazole (+ penicillin)	95	63	43	8.0
Oxytetracycline	97	28	5	16.4

*Among 50 survivors in the original groups.

Note that the frequency of kernicterus in the infants treated with sulfisoxazole is high although the serum bilirubin levels are low as compared to the infants treated with oxytetracycline. There is a paradoxical relationship between bilirubin toxicity and bilirubin serum concentration.

Table 2). Bilirubin as a matter of fact is also bound to the albumin in the interstitial fluid, especially present in the skin. Also there, displacement takes place with similar consequences. In Table 2 there is a remarkable *paradox in the relation* between the *total plasma concentration* of bilirubin and its *toxic action*. The displacement and therewith the shift of bilirubin from plasma to the extravascular compartments causes a strong decrease in the total plasma concentration and a concomitant increase in the toxic effect of bilirubin. Under normal circumstances, as a rule reduction in plasma concentration will imply a reduction in (toxic) action and an increase in plasma concentration will imply an increase there in. If the free, the "active", concentration of bilirubin is taken into account this holds true also in the case of a displacement of bilirubin. The increased toxicity, the kernicterus, goes hand in hand with a (due to the tissue uptake) moderate increase in the free plasma concentration, although the total plasma concentration is reduced.

For certain drugs, for instance phenytoin, a tremendous variation is observed in the plasma concentrations reached in the patients after certain dosages of the drug (Fig. 2) (28). Part of this variation is due to differences in the drug-metabolizing capacity of the patients with regard to phenytoin (29). Since, however, the drug is bound to albumin for about 99%, also variations in albumin concentration are a factor. This becomes clear, if one compares the correlation between *total* plasma concentration of phenytoin and the occurrence of toxic responses in the patients and the correlation for the concentration of the drug in the *unbound* form in the plasma and the occurrence of toxic effects (Fig. 3) (30). This implies that strictly taken measurement of the concentration of the unbound drug would give a better indicator for the control of therapy. In those cases that a correlation between total plasma concentration and response does not exist (31) the concentration of the unbound drug may give a more consistent picture. Interestingly, it turns out that the concentration of a drug in saliva is about the same as the free concentration in plasma and therewith in the extracellular fluid, and that there is a simple linear correlation between these concentrations (Fig. 4) (32). Such relations are reported for a variety of drugs (33, 34). Thus measurement of the drug concentration in saliva may be considered for therapeutic monitoring with as an extra advantage that no venous puncture is required. Since the saliva concentrations for strongly albumin-bound agents are much lower than the (total) plasma concentrations particularly sensitive methods for the determination in saliva may be required.

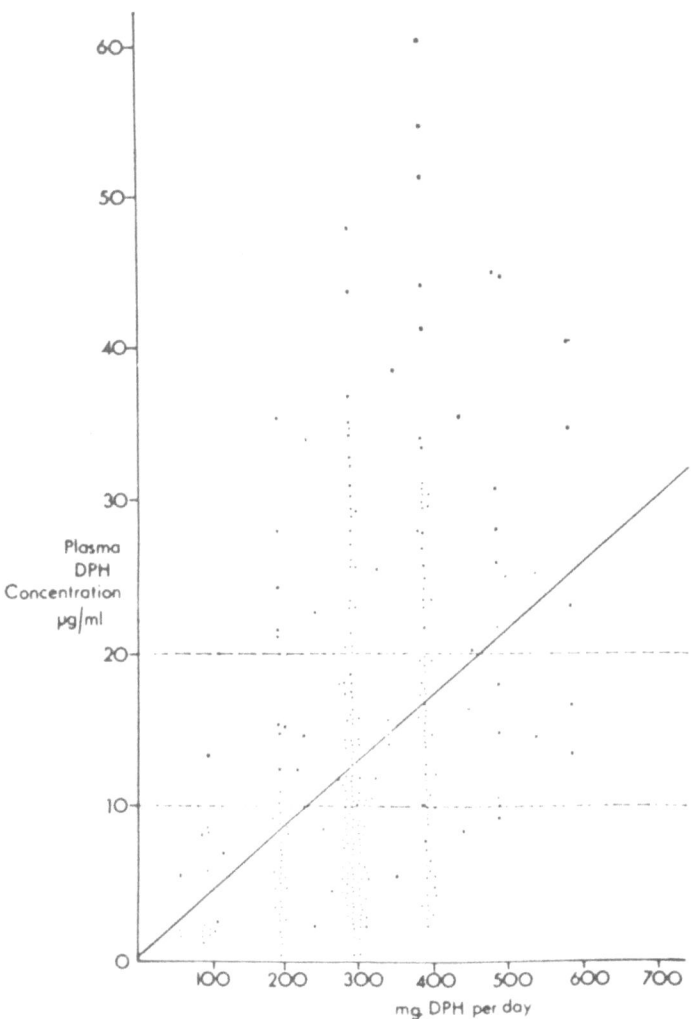

Fig. 2. Steady state plasma concentration of DPH (phenytoin) as a function of the dose measured in 292 patients. Note the tremendous scatter of the values (total plasma concentrations) which in part is due to a variation in drug-metabolizing capacity of the patients while further variations in plasma albumin concentration will be a contributive factor (reproduced from reference 28).

The data on albumin – or plasma protein-binding of drugs in the literature as a rule concern the percentage of protein binding. For many, especially more lipophilic compounds values up to 99% binding are not unusual. A lowering of the bound fraction from 99% to 98% or 97% is only a minor

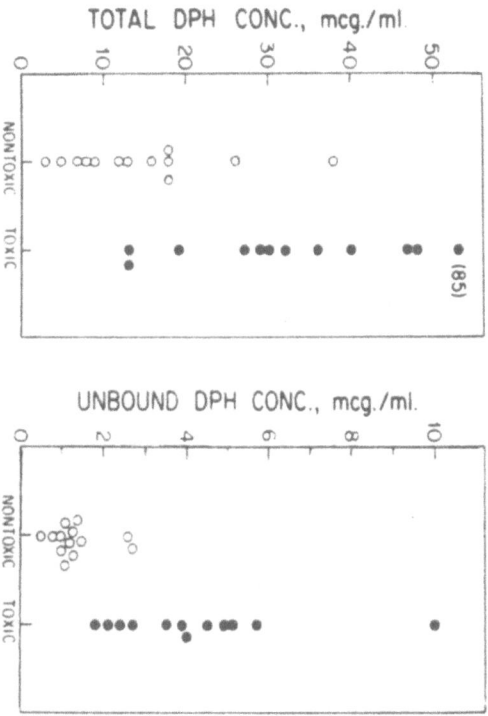

Fig. 3. The relationship between total plasma levels and unbound concentrations in plasma, respectively, for phenytoin (DPH) and toxic action. Note the concentration of the unbound drug is the determinant parameter for toxicity (reproduced from reference 30).

change in the protein binding (see Table 3) (10, 20, 35, 36, 37). However, one should be well aware of the fact that not the concentration of the protein-bound drug but the concentration of the free drug is essential. Both a reduction in the binding due to a displacing drug and a reduction in the binding due to hypoalbuminemia will result in an increase in the free concentration and an increase in the exposure of the tissue cells to the drug. A major part of the fraction normally bound, but now in the unbound form, escapes from the intravascular compartment to the extravascular compartment including the intracellular space where toxic effects can arise then. The rise in the free concentration in plasma, therefore, may be moderate and by no means as large as one would anticipate on basis of the plasma volume only. The total plasma concentration, however, will be appreciably decreased since the quantity of drug in the bound form (strongly bound

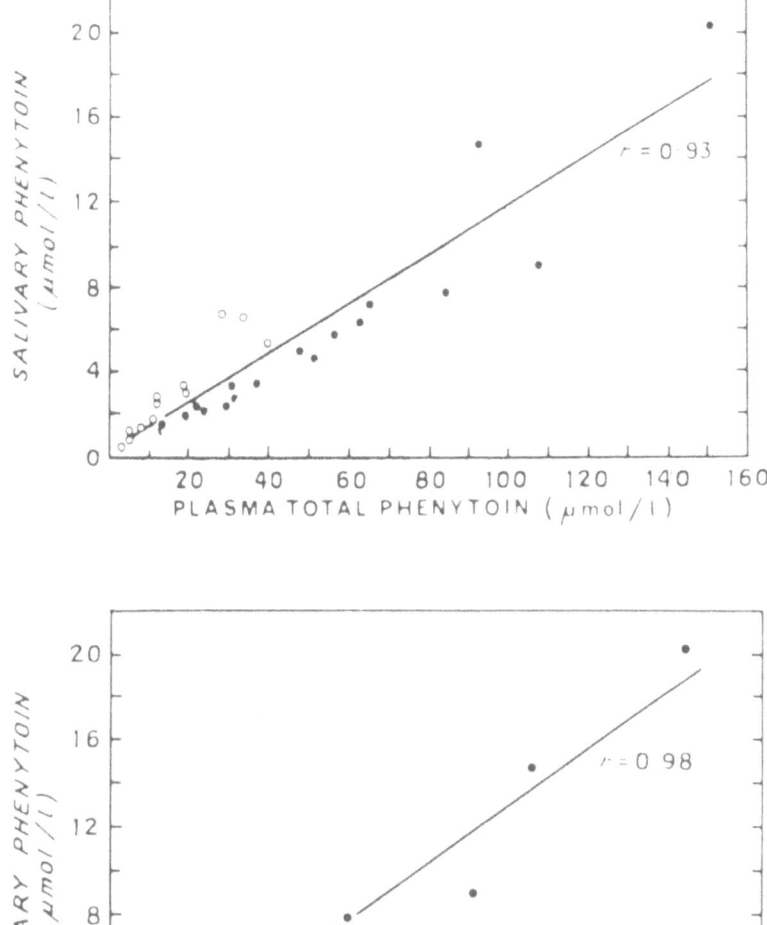

Fig. 4. The relationship between the salivary concentration of phenytoin (diphenylhydantoin) and the concentration of this drug in plasma (● epileptic patients; ○ patients with renal failure). Note that there is a good correlation of the salivary concentration with both the total (Fig. 4a) and the free (Fig. 4b) plasma concentration. The salivary concentration is a good indicator for the free concentration (reproduced from reference 32).

Table 3. Drugs with low free concentrations in human serum due to strong albumin binding (reproduced from references 10, 20, 35, 36, 37, 66)

Drug	Free %	Drug	Free %
Central-Nervous-System		**Renal:**	
Active Drugs:		Probenecid	1
Diazepam	1	Furosemide	3
Amitriptyline	4	Chlorothiazide	5
Imipramine	4	Sulfinpyrazone	5
Chlorpromazine	4	Trichlormethiazide	8
Chlordiazepoxide	5	Ethacrynic acid	10
Nortriptyline	6		
Desipramine	8	**Anti-Infective:**	
Phenytoin	9	Dicloxacillin	2
Methadone	13	Cloxacillin	5
Thiopental	13	Oxacillin	6
		Flucloxacillin	6
Anti-Inflammatory:		Propicillin	13
Fenoprofen	1	Cefazolin	10
Phenylbutazone	1	Doxycycline	7
Indomethacin	3	Nafcillin	10
Oxyphenbutazone	5	Sulfaphenazole	0.1
Salicylic acid	16	Sulfaethidole	4
		Sulfadimethoxine	10
Cardiovascular-Renal:		Sulfamethoxypyridazine	10
Propranolol	6	Sulfisoxazole	16
Diazoxide	9		
Digitoxin	10	**Miscellaneous:**	
Quinidine	11	Methotrexate	6
Hydralazine	13	Clofibrate	10
		Bishydroxycoumarin	0.2
		Warfarin	3
		Tolbutamide	1
		Chlorpropamide	4
		Tolazamide	6

drugs are considered) constituted the major part of the total plasma concentration. The result is a paradoxical situation again, namely a decrease in the total plasma concentration, but an increase in the (total) response (23). It is the increase in the free concentration of the drug and the concomitant shift to the tissues that count, however. Table 4 gives as an example of this phenomenon the displacement of the anticoagulant warfarin by phenylbutazone (38).

In considering the therapeutic plasma concentration ranges from the literature (Table 5) (39, 40, 41) one should take into account the influence

Table 4. The prothrombin activity in plasma as a function of the plasma warfarin concentration and the changes therein as a result of a combination of warfarin with phenylbutazone (reproduced from reference 38)

Dose of warfarin mg/day	Dose of phenylbutazone mg/day	Prothrombin activity* % of normal	Plasma concentration warfarin* mg/l	N
0	0	67.0 ± 5.3	0	17
145	0	27.1 ± 4.2	55.3 ± 6.0	20
50–60	0	68.0 ± 13.4	23.0 ± 3.7	21
55	400	22.8 ± 1.6	9.6 ± 0.7	5

* Mean ± S.D.
N = Number of determinations

Note that with warfarin 50–60 mg alone, there is no effect on the prothrombin activity at a plasma concentration of about 23 mg/liter while with the combination of warfarin and phenylbutazone there is a strong effect on prothrombin activity although the plasma concentration is much lower than with warfarin alone. There is a paradoxical relationship between the change in plasma concentration and the response.

of decreases in the plasma albumin concentration and of displacement of the drug from albumin by a second one. For patients with a hypoalbuminemia, for highly albumin-bound drugs, the "standard" therapeutic ranges in fact may well be toxic ranges.

HYPOALBUMINEMIA AND DRUG ACTION

What consequences can be expected from hypoalbuminemia for drug action? There are quite a number of diseases (42, 43, 44, 45) in which the albumin concentration in plasma is lowered. Casey (46) reports that in a search among 23,000 hospitalized patients 18% had hypoalbuminemia. Generally, there is a concomitant decrease in the albumin concentration in the interstitial compartment. Clinical observations show that indeed in patients with hypoalbuminemia the frequency of side effects with certain drugs is significantly higher than in patients with normal albumin levels. Examples are given in Table 6 (47), Table 7 (48) and Table 8 (49). Similarly with clofibrate in patients with plasma albumin lower than 3 g/100 ml, a much higher incidence of side effects is reported than for patients with normal albumin levels (41). One should be careful, however, in relating the increased incidence of side effects too easily or solely to a decrease in plasma albumin levels.

Table 5. Usual range of therapeutic serum concentrations of drugs (reproduced from references 39, 40, 41)

Drug	Usual therapeutic range
Cardiovascular drugs:	
Digoxin	1–2 ng/ml
Digitoxin	10–25 ng/ml
Quinidine	2–4 μg/ml
Procainamide	4–8 μg/ml
Lidocaine	2–4 μg/ml
Propranolol	20–50 ng/ml
Theophylline	10–20 μg/ml
Antiepileptic drugs:	
Phenytoin	10–20 μg/ml
Phenobarbitone	15–30 μg/ml
Primidone	5–10 μg/ml
Ethosuximide	40–80 μg/ml
N-Desmethylmethsuximide	10–40 μg/ml
Psychoactive drugs:	
Lithium	0.5–1.5 mEq/l
Diazepam	0.5–2.5 μg/ml
Amitriptyline	100–200 ng/ml
Nortriptyline	50–150 ng/ml
Miscellaneous:	
Salicylates*	150–300 μg/ml
Phenylbutazone	± 100 μg/ml
Tolbutamide	53–96 μg/ml
Chlorpropamide	30–140 μg/ml
Probenecid	100–200 μg/ml

For hypoalbuminemic or uremic patients the usual therapeutic range overlaps with or is equal to the toxic range, especially for drugs with a high degree of protein binding (Table 3).
* Used as antirheumatic.

Table 6. Adverse reactions to phenytoin in relation to serum albumin levels (reproduced from reference 47)

Serum albumin (g per 100 ml)	Number of patients exposed	Per cent reactions
< 2.5	30	13.3
2.5–2.9	58	10.3
3.0–3.4	75	6.7
3.5–3.9	60	5.0
≧ 4.0	99	1.0

Note that for patients with low serum albumin levels the incidence of adverse reactions is increased.

Table 7. Adverse reactions to prednisone in relation to the dose and the serum albumin level (reproduced from reference 48)

Mean daily dose mg	Serum albumin g/100 ml	Number of patients	Per cent with side effects
1–25	≤2.5	11	9
	≥2.6	84	12
25–50	≤2.5	11	36
	≥2.6	71	14
>50	≤2.5	13	62
	≥2.6	50	20

Note that for patients with low serum albumin levels the incidence of adverse reactions is increased.

Table 8. Adverse reactions to diazepam in relation to serum albumin levels (reproduced from reference 49).

Serum albumin concentration (g/100 ml)	Number of patients exposed	CNS depression (%)
<3.0	281	26 (9.3%)
3.0–3.4	292	25 (8.9%)
3.5–3.9	323	25 (7.7%)
≥4.0	306	9 (2.9%)

Note that patients with low albumin levels have a higher frequency of adverse reactions.

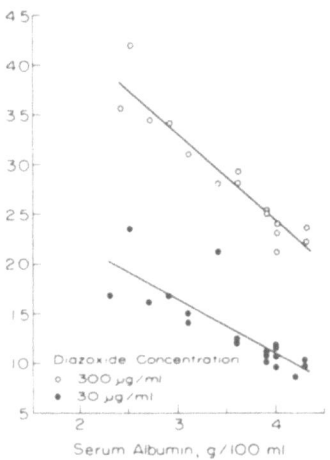

Fig. 5a. The relationship between the free fraction of diazoxide in serum (of a uremic patient) as a function of the albumin concentration. Note the increase in the free fraction at lower albumin concentrations both at lower and higher concentrations of diazoxide (normally highly bound to plasma protein) (reproduced from reference 50).

In the increased frequency of side effects of drugs in patients with low serum-albumin values, various factors may be involved:

a) The lowering of the albumin concentration as such can result in an increase in the free, the active, concentration with a concomitant lowering in the total plasma concentration of the drug (Fig. 5a) (50) and (Fig. 5b) (51). See also Table 9 (61).
b) The hypoalbuminemia may be an aspect of liver or kidney disease and thus imply a decrease in the capacity of these organs for drug elimination. The consequence thereof will be an increase in the total as well as the free plasma concentration of the drug unless the dose is adapted (9, 21, 52, 53, 54, 55, 56, 57).
c) The binding capacity of albumin may be changed under pathological conditions. In uremic patients, for instance, the binding degree especially for the class of weakly acidic drugs to albumin is strongly reduced (21, 58, 59). This implies that the fraction bound to protein and thus the total plasma concentration is decreased and the free concentration is increased. Dialysis of the uremic plasma against charcoal results in a normalization of the binding capacity (Fig. 6) (58). The reduced binding capacity appears to be not the result of conformational changes in the albumin due to the relatively high urea concentrations or of displace-

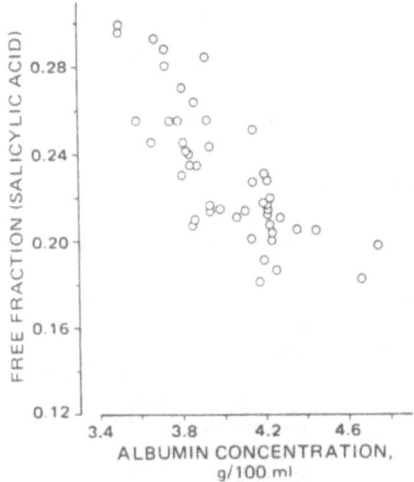

Fig. 5b. The relationship between the free fraction of salicylic acid in serum of human adults (48 individuals) as a function of the albumin concentration. Note the increase in the free fraction at lower albumin concentrations (reproduced from reference 51).

ment by fatty acids, but of a displacement by some hitherto unknown agents (21, 58, 59, 60).

d) In patients with hypoalbuminemia due to liver disease often hyperbilirubinemia will be a concomitant aspect. Unconjugated bilirubin has an extremely high affinity for plasma albumin and thus is very effective in displacing other agents, namely weakly acidic lipophilic drugs (25). The result is an extra decrease in the total plasma concentration and increase in the free, the active concentration of the drug.

In conclusion, under pathological conditions involving hypoalbuminemia, various factors tend to increase the concentration of the free drug and thus to enhance the risk of a relative overdosage and adverse effects, unless the dosage is adapted. For strongly albumin-bound potentially toxic drugs, with a small therapeutic margin, monitoring of the therapy, preferentially on basis of the measurement of the free concentration (e.g. the concentration in saliva) should be considered. This is one of the exceptional situations (62, 63, 64) where monitoring of drug therapy on basis of drug concentrations is rational.

Also with regard to bilirubin itself, hypoalbuminemia is an important factor, since albumin serves as a buffer for unconjugated bilirubin, keeping the free concentration and therewith the tissue and cell concentration low even at high plasma concentrations, not only displacement of bilirubin from albumin by other drugs, but also the reduction in binding capacity in case of hypoalbuminemia will result in a shift of bilirubin to the tissue. In liver disease, hyperbilirubinemia and hypoalbuminemia may well go together. In such cases, at relatively low total plasma bilirubin concentrations (a result of the hypoalbuminemia) a relatively high degree of "tissue jaundice" may be expected.

Table 9. Plasma albumin concentration and drug-albumin binding (reproduced from reference 61)

Drug	Healthy indiv. unbound fraction ($\%$)	Patients disease	albumin conc. (g/100 ml)	unbound fraction ($\%$)
Triamterene	19.3	Liver disease	2.8	33.0
Quinidine	14.1	Liver disease	2.2	41.5
Phenytoin	10.1	Nephrosis	2.3	19.2
Frusemide	2.3	Nephrosis	1.3	6.3
Clofibrate	3.6	Nephrosis	2.2	11.0
Diazoxide	9.9	Uraemia	3.5	13.3

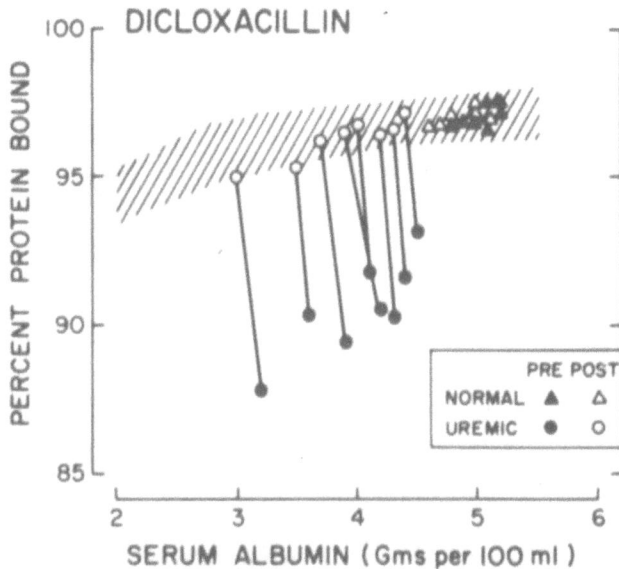

Fig. 6. The protein binding of dicloxacillin in serum at different albumin concentrations in six normal (▲) and eight uremic (●) patients. Note: the protein binding in the uremic patients is very low as compared to that in the normal patients. After treatment of the serum with charcoal (△ and ○ respectively) the protein binding is normalized, but as expected still dependent on the serum albumin concentration (reproduced from reference 58).

A QUANTITATIVE APPROXIMATION

Protein binding of drugs is governed by mass action law. The degree of binding is dependent on the concentrations of both the protein and the drug. Binding curves can be obtained by choosing the drug concentration or the protein concentration as a variable. In both cases the classical type of saturation curve is obtained. For highly bound drugs a small percentual change in the degree of binding in the saturation range has a great influence on the concentration of the unbound drug. A decrease of, for instance, 99% binding to 97% binding, which implies a 2% change, in a closed system has as a consequence that the unbound fraction is triplicated.

Figs. 7 and 8 give binding curves for the case of a constant albumin concentration and different drug concentrations and for the case of a constant drug concentration and different albumin concentrations. As a matter of fact the drug-albumin binding also depends on the affinity between drug and albumin. Fig. 9 gives an example of such a relationship (21, 65).

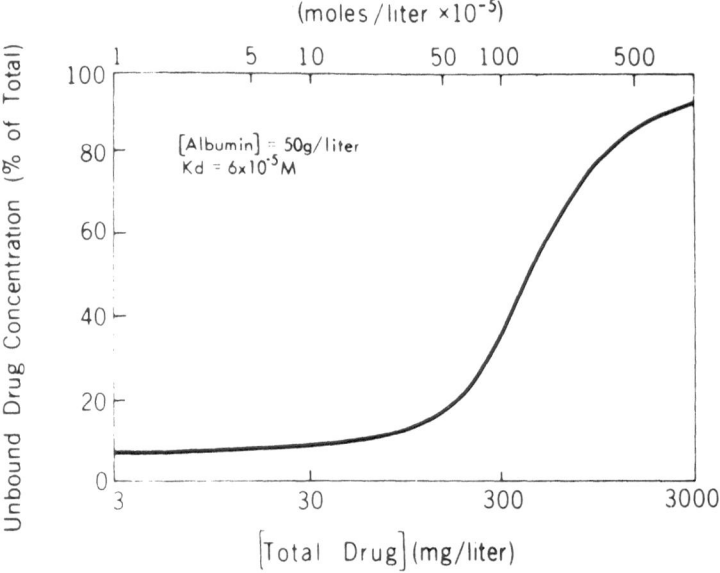

Fig. 7. The influence of changes in total drug concentration on drug-albumin binding at a constant albumin concentration (reproduced from reference 64).

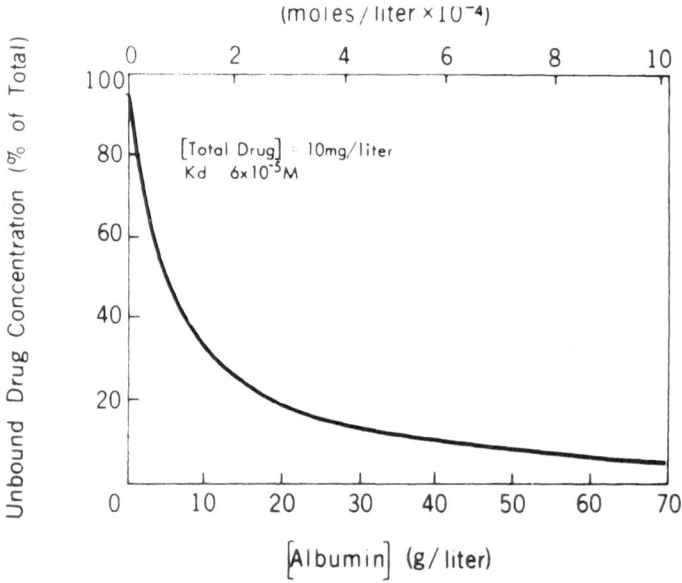

Fig. 8. The influence of changes in the albumin concentration on drug-albumin binding at a constant total drug concentration (reproduced from reference 64).

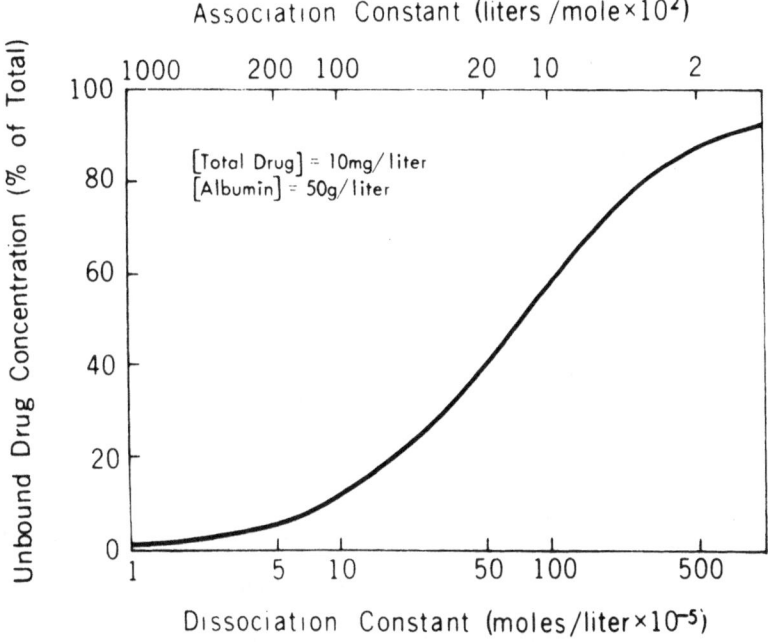

Fig. 9. The influence of changes in the affinity of the drug to albumin on drug-albumin binding at a constant albumin concentration and a constant total drug concentration (reproduced from reference 64).

Many drugs, especially acidic compounds, find one or two high affinity binding sites on each albumin molecule, so that one molar equivalent of plasma albumin can bind one or two moles of the drug. The maximal quantity of a drug with a molecular weight of 300 to be bound to 40 g albumin – assumed to have one binding site – would be 180 mg. If the total quantity of intravascular plus interstitial albumin (270 g) is taken into account and all binding sites are assumed to be available, which implies an absence of competing endulgeous agents, then for drugs with an appreciable affinity (dissociation constant $\leq 10^{-1}$) for albumin, saturation of the albumin is approached with dosages of 400–800 mg. Since a reduction of the albumin concentration to 50% of normal also implies a reduction of the binding capacity to 50%, and as a rule not all binding sites are readily available, increases in the unbound fraction of drugs in diseases with hypoalbuminemia as a symptom is not uncommon. Table 9 (61) gives examples.

As long as with the dose applied, the fraction of the albumin occupied by the drug is small, because of a low dose or a low affinity to albumin, sufficient binding capacity remains available to buffer largely the changes in the free concentration of the drug brought about by reduction in the albumin concentration.

For a detailed discussion of the quantitative and theoretical aspects the reader is referred to the literature (11, 19, 21, 41, 43).

REFERENCES

1. Oratz M, Rothschild MA, Schreiber SS: Albumin-Osmotic Function. In: Albumin Structure, Function and Uses, first edition, VM Rosenoer, M Oratz, MA Rothschild (eds), Oxford, Pergamon Press, 1977, pp 275–282.
2. Ehrnebo M, Agurell S, Jalling B, et al: Age differences in drug binding by plasma proteins: studies on human foetuses, neonates, and adults. Eur J Clin Pharmacol 3: 189–193, 1971.
3. Brodie BB, Maickel RP: Comparative biochemistry of drug metabolism. Proceedings of the First International Pharmacological Meeting 6, August 22–25, 1961. Oxford, Pergamon Press, 1962, pp 299–324.
4. Williams RT: Comparative patterns of drug metabolism. Federation Proceedings 26:1029–1039, 1967.
5. Dewaide JH: Metabolism of Xenobiotics. Thesis University Nijmegen, Nijmegen, Drukkerij Leijn, 1971, pp 83–97.
6. Ariëns EJ, Simonis AM, Offermeier J: Introduction to General Toxicology. New York, Academic Press, 1976, pp 44–79.
7. Remmer H, Casals J: Die Steigerung der Albuminsynthese durch Phenobarbital. Naunyn Schmiedebergs Arch Pharmacol 269:455–456, 1971.
8. Bridges JW, Wilson, AGE: Drug-serum protein interactions and their biological significance. In: Progress in Drug Metabolism, 1, JW Bridges, LF Chasseaud (eds), London, John Wiley and Sons, 1976, pp 193–247.
9. Vallner JJ: Binding of drugs by albumin and plasma protein. J Pharm Sci 66: 447–465, 1977.
10. Curry S: Drug Disposition and Pharmacokinetics. London, Blackwell Scient Publ, 1977, pp 78–91.
11. Briggs M, Briggs M: The chemistry and metabolism of drugs and toxins. London, William Heinemann Medical Books Ltd, 1974, pp 116–126.
12. Henderson PTh: Development and maturation of drug-metabolizing enzymes. Eur J Drug Metabolism and Pharmacokinetics, 1977.
13. Klinger W: Biotransformation in der Leber. In: Entwicklungspharmakologie, H Ankermann (ed), Stuttgart, Gustav Fischer Verlag, 1974, pp 51–126.
14. Sjöqvist F, Bertilsson L: Plasma Concentrations of Drugs and Pharmacological Response in Man. In: Biological Effects of Drugs in Relation to their Plasma Concentrations, DS Davies, BNC Prichard (eds), London, MacMillan Press Ltd, 1973, pp 26–40.
15. Vesell ES: Relationship between drug distribution and therapeutic effects in man. Annu Rev Pharmacol 14:249–270, 1974.
16. Zacest R, Koch-Weser J: Relation of hydralazine plasma concentration to dosage and hypotensive action. Clin Pharmacol Ther 13:420–425, 1972.
17. Lyle WH, Braithwaite RA, Brooks PW, et al: Plasma concentration of nortriptyline as a guide to treatment. Postgraduate Medical Journal 50:282–287, 1974.
18. Gribnau TCJ: Coupling of effector-molecules to solid supports. Thesis University Nijmegen, Nijmegen, Drukkerij van Mameren, 1977, pp 150–153.

19. Jusko WJ, Gretch M: Plasma and tissue protein binding of drugs in pharmacokinetics. Drug Metabolism Reviews 5(1):43–118, 1976.
20. Koch-Weser J, Sellers EM: Binding of drugs to serum albumin (part II). N Engl J Med 294:526–531, 1976.
21. Sellers EM, Koch-Weser J: Clinical implications of drug-albumin interaction. In: Albumin Structure, Function and Uses, first edition, VM Rosenoer, M Oratz, MA Rothschild (eds) Oxford, Pergamon Press, 1977, pp 159–182.
22. Martin EW: Drug Interactions. In: Hazards of Medication, Philadelphia, JB Lippincott Company, 1971, pp 378–875.
23. Ariëns EJ, Simonis AM: Drug interactions resulting in loss of action. In: Clinical Effects of interaction between drugs, LE Cluff, JC Petrie (eds), Amsterdam, Excerpta Medica, 1974, pp 69–102.
24. Ariëns EJ, Simonis AM: The mechanisms of adverse drug reactions. In: Drug-Induced Diseases, 4, L Meyler, HM Peck (eds) Amsterdam, Excerpta Medica, 1972, pp 110–178.
25. Odell GB: Influence of binding on the toxicity of bilirubin. Ann NY Acad Sci 226:225–237, 1973.
26. Silverman WA, Andersen DH, Blanc WA, et al: A difference in mortality rate and incidence of kernicterus among premature infants allotted to two prophylactic antibacterial regimens. Pediatrics 18:614–625, 1956.
27. Koslowski H, Menzel K, Braun W: In vitro-Untersuchungen zum Medikamenteneinfluss auf die Albumin-Bilirubin-Bindung. Kinderärztl Prax 43:66–72, 1975.
28. Eadie MJ, Tyrer JH: Anticonvulsant Therapy. Edinburgh and London, Churchill Livingstone, 1974, pp. 43–59.
29. Richens A, Dunlop, A: Serum-phenytoin levels in management of epilepsy. Lancet 2:247–248, 1975.
30. Booker HE, Darcey B: Serum concentrations of free diphenylhydantoin and their relationship to clinical intoxication. Epilepsia 14:177–184, 1973.
31. Perrier D, Gibaldi M: Drug Concentrations in the Plasma as an Index of Pharmacologic Effect. J Clin Pharmacol 14:415–417, 1974.
32. Reynolds F, Jones NF, Ziroyanis PN, et al: Salivary phenytoin concentrations in epilepsy and in chronic renal failure. Lancet 2:384–386, 1976.
33. Speirs CF: Oral absorption and secretion of drugs. Br J Clin Pharmac 4:97–100, 1977.
34. Feller K, Le Petit G: On the distribution of drugs in saliva and blood plasma. Int J Clin Pharmacol 15:468–469, 1977.
35. Koch-Weser J: Drug interactions in cardiovascular therapy. Amer Heart J 90:93–116, 1975.
36. Barza M, Weinstein L: Pharmacokinetics of the penicillins in man. Clinical Pharmacokinetics 1:297–308, 1976.
37. Moellering RC, Swartz MN: The newer cephalosporins. N Engl J Med 294:24–28, 1976.
38. Aggeler PM, O'Reilly RA, Leong L. et al: Potentiation of anticoagulant effect of warfarin by phenylbutazone. N Engl J Med 276:496–501, 1967.
39. Sjöqvist F: Clinical Use of drug plasma level determinations. In: The Year Book of Drug Therapy, DL Azarnoff (ed), Chicago, Year Book Medical Publishers, Inc., 1977, pp 13–20.
40. Atkinson AJ: Individualization of anticonvulsant therapy. Med Clin North Am 58:1037–1049, 1974.
41. Wagner JG: Fundamentals of Clinical Pharmacokinetics, first edition, Hamilton, Drug Intelligence Publications, 1975, pp 46–52.
42. van Tongeren JHM: Causes of hypoalbuminemia. This volume.
43. Jusko WJ: Pharmacokinetics in disease states changing protein binding. In: The Effect

of Disease States on Drug Pharmacokinetics, LZ Benet (ed), Washington, American Pharmaceutical Association, 1976, pp 99–123.

44. Fabre J, Ohr I: Drug selection and dosage in renal insufficiency. In: Ergebnisse der Inneren Medizin und Kinderheilkunde, 34, P Frick, GA von Harnack, GA Martini, A Prader, R Schoen, HP Wolff (eds), Berlin, Springer-Verlag, 1974, pp 46–93.

45. Boobis SW: Alteration of plasma albumin in relation to decreased drug binding in uremia. Clin Pharmacol Ther 22:147–153, 1977.

46. Casey AE, Gilbert FE, Copeland H, et al: Albumin, alpha 1, 2, beta and gamma globulin in cancer and other diseases. South Med J 66:179–185, 1973.

47. Boston Collaborative Drug Surveillance Program: Diphenylhydantoin side effects and serum albumin levels. Clin Pharmacol Ther 14:529–532, 1973.

48. Lewis GP, Jusko WJ, Burke ChW, et al: Prednisone side-effects and serum-protein levels. Lancet II:778–781, 1971.

49. Greenblatt DJ, Koch-Weser J: Clinical toxicity of chlordiazepoxide and diazepam in relation to serum albumin concentration: a report from the Boston Collaborative Drug Surveillance Program. Eur J Clin Pharmacol 7:259–262, 1974.

50. O'Malley K, Velasco M, Pruitt A, et al: Decreased plasma protein binding of diazoxide in uremia. Clin Pharmacol Ther 18:53–58, 1975.

51. Yacobi A, Levy G: Intraindividual relationships between serum protein binding of drugs in normal human subjects, patients with impaired renal function, and rats. J Pharm Sci 66:1285–1287, 1977.

52. Rowland M, Blaschke TF, Meffin PJ, et al: Pharmacokinetics in disease states modifying hepatic and metabolic function. In: The Effect of Disease States on Drug Pharmacokinetics, LZ Benet (ed), Washington, American Pharmaceutical Association, 1976, pp 53–76.

53. Welling PG, Craig WA: Pharmacokinetics in disease states modifying renal function. In: The Effect of Disease States on Drug Pharmacokinetics, LZ Benet (ed), Washington, American Pharmaceutical Association, 1976, pp 155–188.

54. Reidenberg MM: Mechanisms of Excretion of Drugs. In: Renal Function and Drug Action, Philadelphia, WB Saunders Company, 1971, pp 5–17.

55. Bennett WM, Singer I, Coggins CH: A practical guide to drug usage in adult patients with impaired renal function. JAMA 214:1468–1475, 1970.

56. Bennett WM, Singer I, Coggins CH: Guide to drug usage in adult patients with impaired renal function. JAMA 223:991–997, 1973.

57. Klotz U: Influence of liver disease on the elimination of drugs. Eur J Drug Metabolism Pharmacokinetics 1:129–140, 1976.

58. Craig WA, Evenson MA, Sarver KP, et al: Correction of protein binding defect in uremic sera by charcoal treatment. J Lab Clin Med 87:637–647, 1976.

59. Bridgman JF, Rosen SM, Thorp JM: Complications during clofibrate treatment of nephrotic-syndrome hyperlipoproteinaemia. Lancet, II:506–509, 1972.

60. Sjöholm I, Kober A, Odar-Cederlöf I, et al: Protein binding of drugs in uremic and normal serum: the role of endogenous binding inhibitors. Biochem Pharmacol 25:1205–1213, 1976.

61. Gugler R, Azarnoff DL: Drug protein binding and the nephrotic syndrome. Clin Pharmacokin 1:25–35, 1976.

62. Dollery CT: When ought we to measure plasma concentrations in clinical practice? In: Biological Effects of Drugs in relation to Their Plasma Concentrations, DS Davies, BNC Prichard (eds), London, MacMillan Press, 1973, pp 241–245.

63. Werner M, Sutherland EW, Abramson FP: Concepts for the rational selection of assays to be used in monitoring therapeutic drugs. Clin Chem 21, 1368–1371, 1975.

64. Riegelman S, Sadee W: Which drugs can and should be monitored today and tomorrow?

In: Clinical Pharmacokinetics, Symposium October 1974, G Levy (ed), Washington, American Pharmaceutical Association, 1974, pp 169–179.
65. Koch-Weser J, Sellers EM: Binding of drugs to serum albumin (part 1). N Engl J Med 294:311–315, 1976.
66. Schröder E, Rufer C, Schmiecher R: Arzneimittel III: Chemotherapeutica. Stuttgart, Georg Thieme Verlag, 1976, pp 57–59.

11. Preparation and control of serum albumin

H.W. KRIJNEN

In the Central Laboratory of the Netherlands Red Cross Blood Transfusion Service, human serum albumin is isolated from venous plasma obtained by the centrifugal separation of the cell components and plasma from human whole blood, collected either in ACD-(acid citrate dextrose) or CPD-(citrate phosphate dextrose) anticoagulant solutions.

Among the criterias for donor selection, the absence of HBsAg (Hepatitis B surface Antigen) is of great importance.

The main reasons of the isolation of plasma proteins (among them albumin) for clinical use are the following:

1. to utilize the valuable human plasma as optimally as possible,
2. to reduce the side effects,
3. to obtain concentrated solution of particular component,
4. to increase the stability of the protein,
5. to reduce the risk of HBsAg transmission.

Various methods are available to separate plasma proteins such as: electrophoresis, ultracentrifugation, precipitation, chromatography, gelfiltration and ultrafiltration. However, for large scale operations, precipitation techniques in combination with chromatography, gelfiltration and ultra filtration are mostly applied.

Although simplified to a great extent, the Cohn system is still widely used for the precipitation of different plasma proteins, with the aid of ethanol as a precipitating agent. In that system, 5 variables are exploited to obtain the precipitation of specific proteins: a. ethanol concentration (8–40%), b. temperature ($-3°$ to $-6°C$), c. pH (4.5–7.4), d. protein concentration, e. ionic strength.

The 20% Albumin solution and the pasteurized plasma protein solution, as supplied by the Central Laboratory of the Netherlands Red Cross Blood

Transfusion Service, are isolated as described in the fractionation scheme (Fig. 1).

After separation by centrifugation the precipitated proteins are freeze dried to remove residual ethanol and water. The albumin containing powders are dissolved to the desired protein concentration and sterilized by filtration. By the addition of sodium caprylate and/or sodium mandelate as albumin stabilizers, the final albumin- and plasma protein solution in containers, can be heated for 10 hrs. at 60°C to inactivate the causative agent of serum hepatitis.

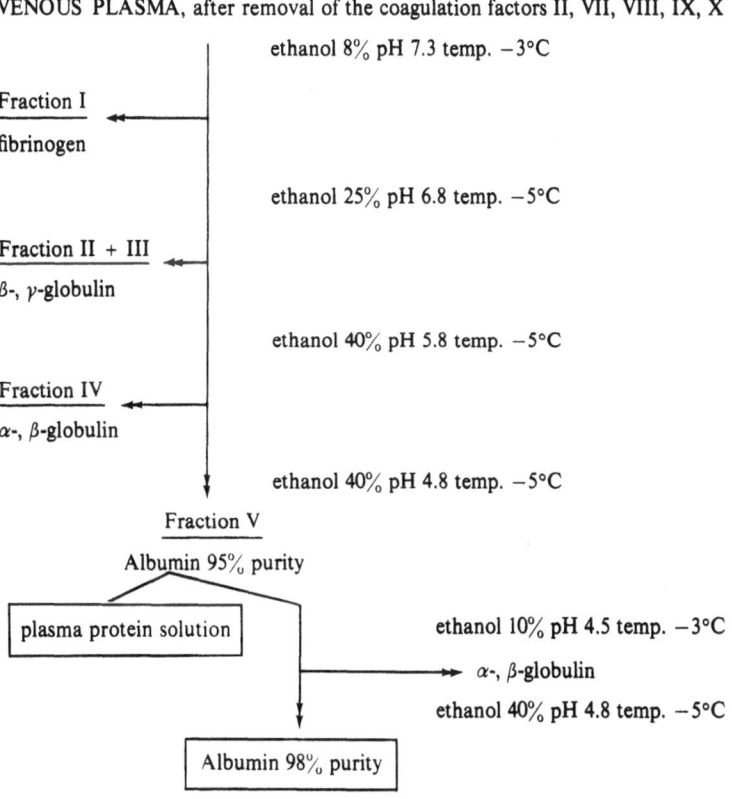

VENOUS PLASMA, after removal of the coagulation factors II, VII, VIII, IX, X

ethanol 8% pH 7.3 temp. −3°C

Fraction I

fibrinogen

ethanol 25% pH 6.8 temp. −5°C

Fraction II + III

β-, γ-globulin

ethanol 40% pH 5.8 temp. −5°C

Fraction IV

α-, β-globulin

ethanol 40% pH 4.8 temp. −5°C

Fraction V

Albumin 95% purity

plasma protein solution

ethanol 10% pH 4.5 temp. −3°C

α-, β-globulin

ethanol 40% pH 4.8 temp. −5°C

Albumin 98% purity

Fig. 1. Fractionation scheme of albumin and plasma protein solution.

The composition of the pasteurized plasma protein solution is:

total protein   38 g per liter
albumin   36 g per liter
dextrose   30 g per liter
sodium   1.3–1.6 g per liter (56–70 mmol./liter)
potassium   < 78 mg per liter (2 mmol./liter)
caprylate   0.6 g per liter (4 mmol./liter)

The composition of the 20% albumin solution is:

total protein   200 g per liter
albumin   195 g per liter
sodium   < 3.5 g per liter (< 153 mmol./liter)
potassium   < 78 mg per liter (< 2 mmol./liter)
caprylate   2.86 g per liter (20 mmol./liter)
mandelate   3.02 g per liter (20 mmol./liter)

12. Utilization pattern of plasma protein and albumin

Y.A. Hekster, R.W.M.M. Langenhoff, L.J.B.
Zuidgeest, J.C.L.H. Benneker and
E. van der Kleijn

INTRODUCTION

The steep increase in the use of expensive groups of drugs, such as antibiotics, antineoplastic agents and blood products has led to a rapid increase in costs of drug therapy (1) and of the proportion of medical supplies
to the total hospital drug budget (2).

Data on total drug cost, as shown in Fig. 1, indicate that this steep increase occurred especially after 1974. The extension of the Intensive Care
and Coronary Care units in 1974 has contributed to the rapid increase in
cost in 1975. These two wards with 15 beds, accounted for about 20% of the
total drug budget in the period of 1974–1976 (1).

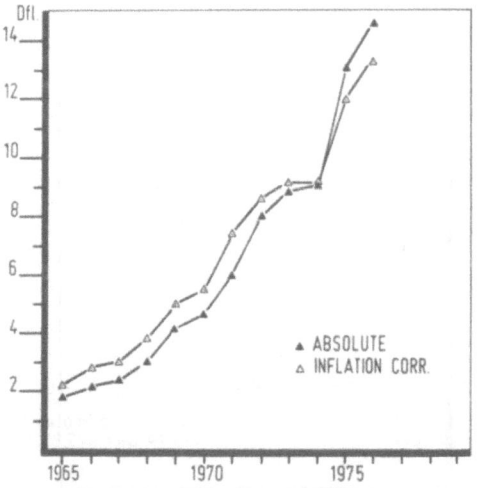

Fig. 1. Costs of drug therapy per day of hospitalization.

The relative high contribution of albumin to the total drug budget can be seen in Fig. 2. Two main blood products: albumin 20% and plasma protein fraction 3.8% (PPF), account for about 20% of total drug expenditure.

INCREASE OF ALBUMIN USE

Fig. 3 reveals the data on the use of PPF and albumin 20%. From these data, a total use of albumin is calculated according to albumin contents of these formulations. A rapid increase can be observed. As prices have not increased since 1974, the economical pattern also reflects the increase in units of use (Fig. 4). These data have alerted those responsible for the pre-scription, distribution and management of drugs. A working committee was instituted to collect and review data on the actual use of albumin per patient during admission to the hospital.

ALBUMIN USE ON THE WARD

Investigations were carried out to determine the main users of these pro-ducts from January to July 1977. It turned out that only a few wards account

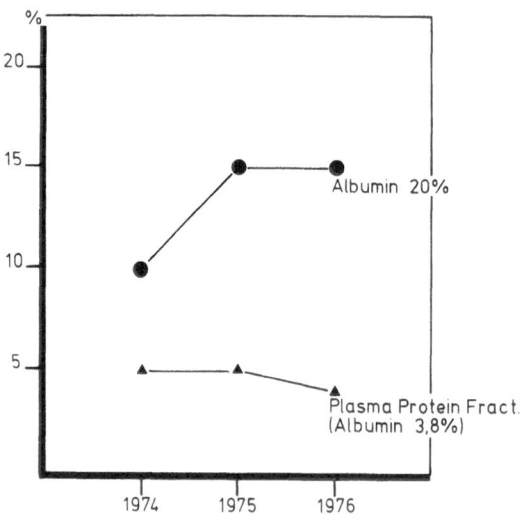

Fig. 2. Percentage of albumin cost to total drug cost.

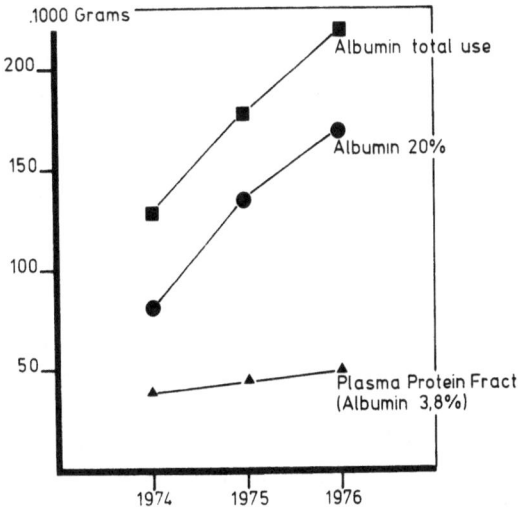

Fig. 3. Clinical use of albumin per year.

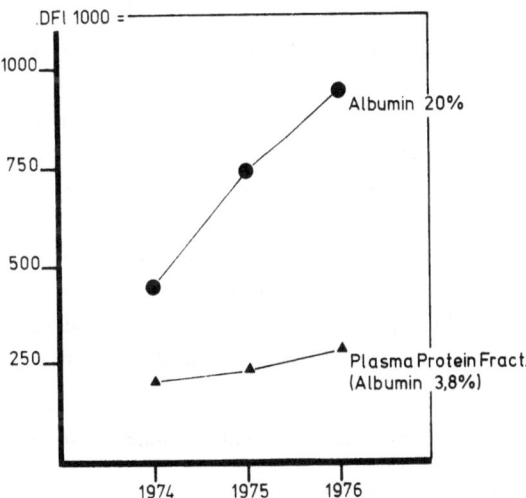

Fig. 4. Economics of albumin use.

for 74.3% of total albumin turnover in this hospital (Table 1). The contribution of the department of anaesthesiology, however, was not open for investigation for individual use per patient. So, only those data with clear

Table 1. Contribution of individual ward/unit on albumin use

Ward	Contribution to total albumin use	
	Albumin 20%	PPF
Intensive care unit	21.3%	17.3
Coronary care unit	20.8%	14.1
Surgery (male)	12.3%	3.7
Surgery (female)	4.7%	3.9
Gastroenterology	7.0%	5.5
Anaesthesiology	8.2%	18.3
Total	74.3%	62.8%

information which could be gathered on the use of albumin per individual patient were utilized for analysis. On these wards the number of patients treated with albumin 20% and/or PPF is shown in Table 2.

INDIVIDUAL ALBUMIN USE

The medication record charts of these patients were used to study the utilization pattern on the ward. The actual use per day was calculated for the suppletion period only. The suppletion period was considered as the number of days from the first to the last administration of albumin. The duration of hospitalization would not influence these statistics and this pattern would, therefore, give relevant information on handling of these drugs. Figs. 5, 6, 7, 8 and 9 show the various patterns of albumin use on the wards, studied. On these wards patients were treated with 1–3 units of albumin per day. The protocol for the dosage regimen was rather uniform and irrespective of variation in patients, intensive care unit and coronary

Table 2. Percentage of patients, admitted on different wards, treated with albumin and/or PPF

Ward	Patients admitted	Patients treated with albumin and/or PPF	Percentage
Intensive care unit	101	90	89.1
Coronary care unit	132	94	71.2
Surgery (male)	328	37	11.3
Surgery (female)	280	21	7.5
Gastroenterology	201	13	6.5

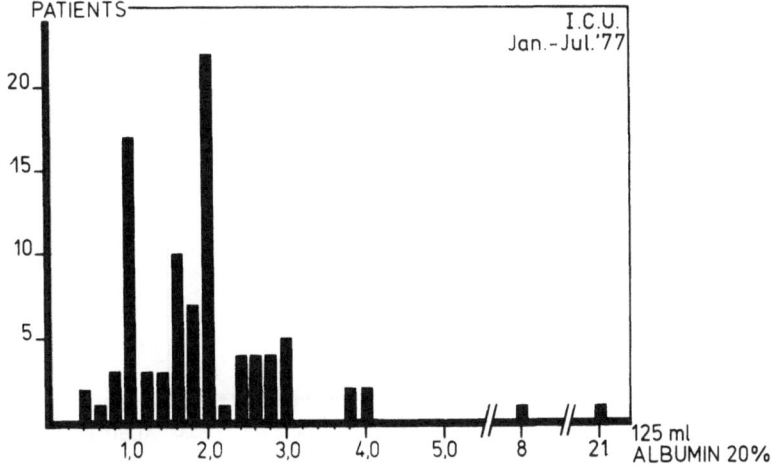

Fig. 5. The utilization pattern of albumin in the intensive care unit. Units albumin per day during suppletion period.

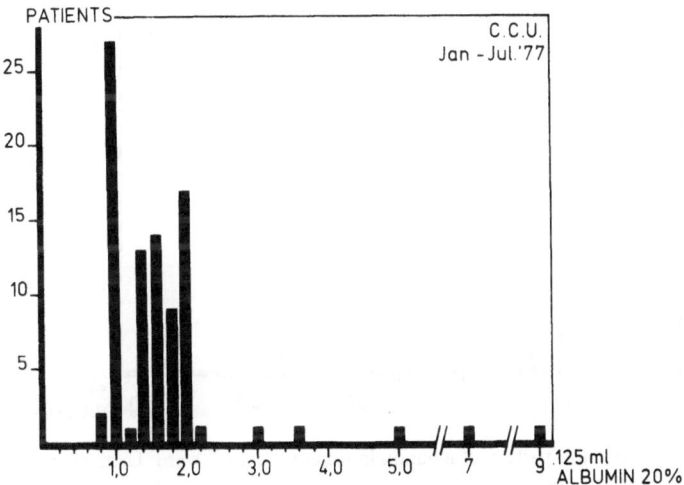

Fig. 6. The utilization pattern of albumin in the coronary care unit. Units albumin per day during suppletion period.

care unit were using these blood products as a routine, this in contrast with the other wards studied (Table 2). However, for further investigation and audit of the proper use based on clinical indications, these data were handed over to the responsible physician.

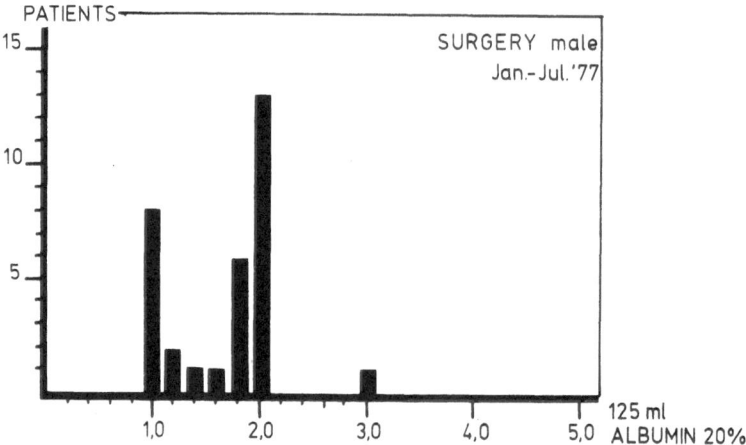

Fig. 7. The utilization pattern of albumin in surgery (male) ward. Units albumin per day during suppletion period.

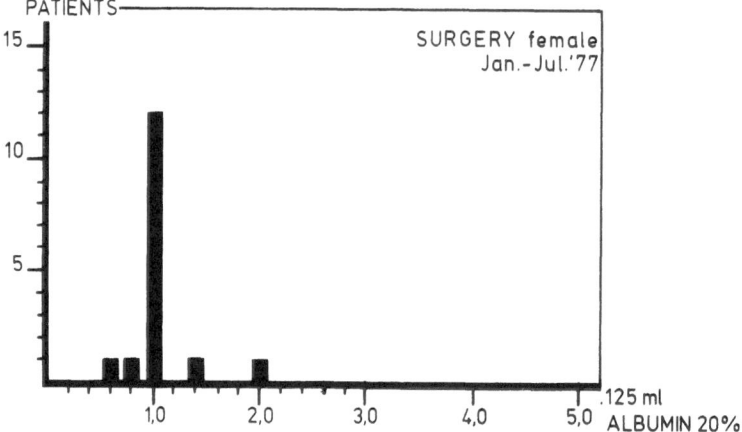

Fig. 8. The utilization pattern of albumin in surgery (female) ward. Units albumin per day during suppletion period.

USE OF ALBUMIN DURING HOSPITALIZATION

If all patients receiving albumin, were categorised based on the number of units of albumin that they received during the hospitalization period, it can be seen in Fig. 10 that about 50% of patients received 1 to 4 units of

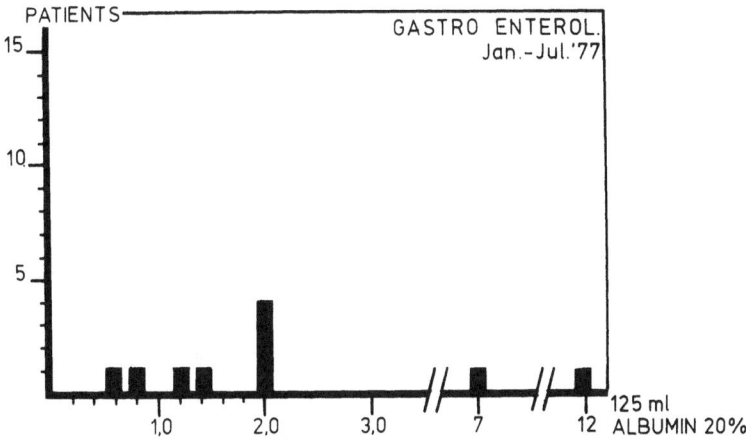

Fig. 9. The utilization pattern ot albumin in the gastroenterology ward. Units albumin per day during suppletion period.

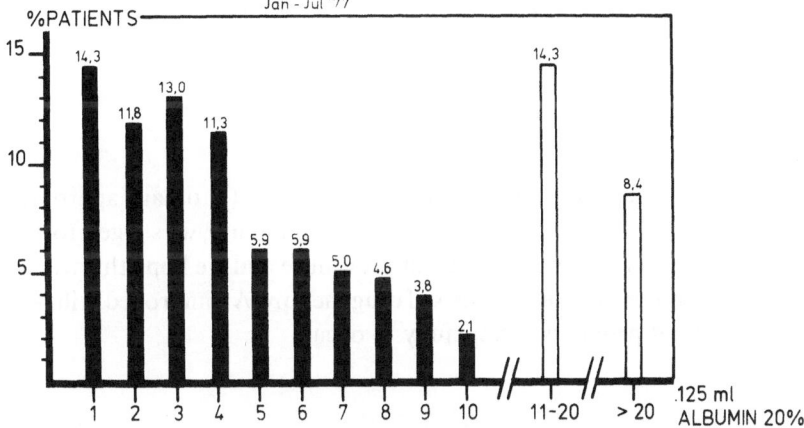

Fig. 10. The overall utilization pattern of albumin (units) from total number of patients (224 patients) studied in St. Radboud Hospital, Jan.–Jul. 1977.

albumin during hospitalization. The usefulness of this number is open for discussion and medical audit (3). The data in Fig. 10, however, show a similar pattern as reported by Lundh et al. from Sweden (4). Nevertheless large differences can be observed between university hospital and general hospital in one country (see appendix, Table 3). Further investigation is

Table 3. Total use of albumin and PPF

	Albumin units (125 ml albumin, 20% = 1 unit)			PPF units (250 ml, PPF = 1 unit)			albumin (kg)		
University hospital	1974	1975	1976	1974	1975	1976	1974	1975	1976
– Amsterdam (Wilh. Gasthuis)	185	695	1410	6064	7618	6278	62	90	95
– Groningen	625	799	2295	no data available			–	–	–*
– Leiden	825	2458	3621	3571	5134	6574	55	110	153
– Maastricht (St. Annadal)	300	585	1160	–	72	252	–	15	31
– Nijmegen (St. Radboud)	3213	5357	6787	4082	4607	5293	119	188	221
– Rotterdam (Dijk-zigt)	781	1029	1029	5526	5400	7920	72	77	101
– Utrecht	135	110	100	2825	3124	4176	30	32	42
General Hospital									
Den Haag	96	504	1168	2636	3532	3164	27	46	59
Leeuwarden (Triotel)		12	92	96	537	468		5	7
Meppel-Hoogeveen	–	–	34	3	24	12	–	–	1
Venlo-Tegelen	68	120	318	1714	886	1118	18	11	19

* From 1-8-'76 till 1-8-'77: 17857 units of PPF.

needed to manage the increase of albumin use. To obtain appropriate guidelines and medical audits concerning albumin use, we suggest to begin with a proper domestic management procedure and we hope this will lead to a reduction in misuse and costs of drug therapy. An improved utilization of these blood products is hopefully to occur.

Table 4. Percentage of total albumin cost to total drug cost

	1974	*1975*	*1976*
University hospital			
– Amsterdam		no data available	
– Groningen		no data available	
– Leiden	13.1	22.2	26.6
– Maastricht	2.3	5.1	8.1
– Nijmegen	15	20	19
– Rotterdam	10.4	9.5	11.6
– Utrecht	5.0	5.0	5.2
General Hospital			
– Den Haag	2.6	4.3	4.0
– Leeuwarden	–	0.4	1.6
– Meppel-Hoogeveen		no data available	
– Venlo-Tegelen	9.4	6.3	7.3

Table 5. Main users (Jan.–June 1977)

	Albumin units (125 ml)	*PPF units* (250 ml)
1. *Rotterdam*		
Intensive care unit	34.6%	21.5%
Surgery	19.5%	–
Internal medicine	17.1%	5.8%
Post operative cardio surgery	–	17.8%
Anaesthesiology	15.1%	28.9%
Other wards	13.8%	26.5%
2. *Venlo-Tegelen*		
Intensive care unit	84%	30%
Surgery	–	24%
Anaesthesiology	–	3%
3. *Leeuwarden*		
Intensive care/coronary care unit	100%	100%
b. *Utrecht*		
Internal medicine	27.2%	27.0%
Intensive care unit (Internal medicine)	60.6%	20.0%
Surgery	1.9%	17.3%
Neurosurgery	4.8%	4.0%
Intensive care unit (surgery)	–	17.0%
Coronary care unit	–	2.9%

APPENDIX

Data from several institutions were collected on our request.
- Table 3 shows data on total use of albumin and PPF (all data converted to 125 ml units of albumin and 250 ml units of PPF).
- Table 4 shows data on the relative part of these two blood products to total drug costs.
- Table 5 gives information on the "main-users" of these blood products in other hospitals.

The high contribution of the intensive care unit in the total use of albumin and PPF in these hospitals is very obvious as has been seen in data collected from our hospital (St. Radboud Hospital).

ACKNOWLEDGEMENT

We gratefully acknowledge the cooperation of Chr. Barrett M.S. (London); Dr. A.M. Berg (Den Haag); Drs. M.H.J. van Gerven (Leiden); Drs. P. Hanff (Venlo); Drs. H.H. Harmsen (Meppel-Hoogeveen); Drs. J.N. Jedema (Leeuwarden); Drs. E.K. Juul Christensen (Groningen); Dr. J.B. Lenstra (Rotterdam); Drs. A.C. van Loenen (Utrecht); Drs. C.W.R. Phaf (Maastricht); Dr. B. Westerholm (Stockholm) and Drs. W.M. de Wit (Amsterdam) for their supply of the information on albumin use in their institutions, as categorised in the appendix.

REFERENCES

1. Hekster YA, Zuidgeest LJB, Hoelen AJ, Bakker JH, van der Kleijn E: Management of hospital drug distribution and utilization. In: Clinical Pharmacy, van der Kleijn E , JR Jonkers (eds), Amsterdam, Elsevier/North Holland Biomedical Press, 79–101, 1977.
2. van der Kleijn E, Okhuijsen-Haarselhorst MACJ, Zuidgeest LJB, Hoelen AJ, Nabuurs AEM: Assortimentsbeheer en gebruik van geneesmiddelen in het St Radboud Ziekenhuis te Nijmegen. Ontwikkeling, onderhoud en handhaving van een ziekenhuis geneesmiddelenformularium en methoden voor geneesmiddelen verzorging. Pharmaceutisch Weekblad, 113:369–388, 1978.
3. Goris RJA: Use and abuse of albumin and plasma protein infusions in acute clinical situations. This book, pp 185–193.
4. Benght L, Grönkvist U, Olsson AM: Behöver man använda Så mycket albumin. In: Läkartidningen, volym 73 (no 14): 1319–1321, 1976.

13. Use and abuse of albumin and plasma-protein infusions in acute clinical situations

R.J.A. GORIS

Standards concerning the use and abuse of antibiotics have been carefully discussed and established (1). Similar standards should also be elaborated to improve the clinical use of albumin and plasma protein infusions. The extensive and careful investigations on albumin use, culminating in the Workshop on Albumin in 1975 (Workshop on Albumin, Feb. 12–13, 1975, National Heart and Lung Institute, National Institute of Health Bethesda Md, U.S.A.), already provided us with a number of guidelines. In this chapter I would like to discuss some standards gathering when or when not to use albumin infusion in acute clinical conditions and the saving of albumin that could have resulted – retrospectively – from the application of these standards in our patients.

Most of us will agree that albumin infusion is not indicated when the serum albumin concentration is 40 g/liter or higher (considered to be as standard 1). In the absence of acute external loss of albumin, there is probably no reason to give albumin more than the intravascular amount in 24 hrs. This amounts to a maximum of 4 units of albumin 20% solution (125 ml/unit) in an adult patient (standard 2). That albumin should not be given to surgical patients with inoperable cancer can also be considered as a general acceptable standard (standard 3). Of course albumin should not be administered if a clear indication is not present (standard 4).

The use of albumin in two major acute clinical situations: the Adult Respiratory Distress Syndrome (ARDS), and shock in high-risk patients should be discussed in more detail.

The Adult Respiratory Distress Syndrome is characterized by decreasing pulmonary compliance and increasing pulmonary edema with a normal or low left atrial pressure. ARDS can not be attributed to shock only, nor to colloid versus crystalloid resuscitation. An additional pulmonary insult is necessary for the occurrence of this syndrome, especially sepsis (2, 3). It has been shown in a consecutive series of intensive care patients, that the combination of peritoneal sepsis and respiratory failure is associated with a high mortality rate (80%), and this group of patients had the lowest serum albumin concentration (mean 23 g/liter) and the lowest compliance (4). In patients with evidence of fat mobilisation, the incidence of pulmonary insufficiency was high if the serum albumin concentration was lower than 28 g/liter (5). Since free fatty acids can cause respiratory distress, and albumin is known to bind fatty acids (6), the use of albumin infusion for supportive therapy in patients with established ARDS seems to be very well motivated, except when standards 1, 2 or 3 hold good. In this latter situation, it is considered to be albumin abuse (standard 5).

Before we discuss the use and abuse of albumin in various shock situations, we have to make clear that there are exceptional events for high-risk patients. Patients older than 70 years or patients with severe intercurrent disease and patients with severe head trauma or pulmonary contusion belong in this high risk group, because in such situations crystalloid resuscitation can bring more hazards than colloid resuscitation. However, if standards 1, 2 or 3 are also present, it has to be considered again as albumin abuse (standard 6).

In the resuscitation of patients in traumatic and hemorrhagic shock, albumin infusion will very likely be the first choice of most people as long as cross-matched blood is not yet available. However, it has convincingly been demonstrated that blood loss can be replaced effectively by adequate amounts of crystalloid solution (7, 8). Previously, it has been demonstrated that progressive hemodilution in dogs–to a hematocrit less than 7% and a plasma protein concentration less than 10 g/liter – does not result in an impairment of blood oxygenation or pulmonary edema. Although there is an increase of body weight by 36% (9) and of lung water by 47%, interstitial edema of this magnitude does not interfere with blood gas exchanges (10). These phenomena can be explained by the fact that the hydrostatic pressure in the pulmonary capillary is approximately three times lower than in the systemic circulation, whereas the oncotic pressure in both is at the same level (6). Moreover, a fall in lymph colloid-osmotic pressure and an increased lymph flow in the lung as found in such a situation can be advantageous for blood gas exchanges (11).

However, in man, crystalloid resuscitation leads to a larger fluid load, a significant rise in body weight, and a significant decrease in serum albumin concentration (12). In preoperative hemodilution, colloid infusion has been proved superior to crystalloid in terms of increasing cardiac output and improving systemic oxygen transport (13). But crystalloid infusion as a temporary substitute for blood loss in severe thoracic trauma (14), and during laparotomy for acute trauma (15), is safe and does not result in a higher incidence of pulmonary edema or postoperative pulmonary insufficiency (15, 16). The intrapulmonary shunt is not increased (17), and a prolonged water retention can not be demonstrated (18). Therefore, it seems reasonable for traumatic and hemorrhagic shock in healthy young patients to start infusion with 3000 ml of crystalloid and 1000 ml of haemacel or dextran solution. This 4-liter infusion volume should allow us time to prepare cross-matched blood. Albumin-containing solutions should not be administered earlier, except in high-risk patients (standard 7).

A similar management program can also be instituted in otherwise healthy patients with septic shock which is recognized in the early stage (standard 8). In this regard, it is interesting to note that administration of pure colloid does not prevent the occurrence of lung edema during septic shock in experimental animals (19). In patients with protracted sepsis due to intraperitoneal infection performing a laparotomy is more life saving than the protracted administration of albumin to support an ailing circulation. As demonstrated in various studies (20, 23), burn-shock can be treated with administration of balanced saline solutions as the sole form of therapy. The administration of isotonic sodium solutions alone (3–4 ml per kg per percent body surface burned) results in a substantial weight gain and edema. Resuscitation with hypertonic alkaline solutions, and no colloid, is accomplished with less fluid intake (1 ml per kg per percent body surface burned), less weight gain, less edema, and with urine output averaging 30 ml per hour (20, 22). The incidence of pulmonary edema has been shown to be significantly reduced in the hypertonic saline group as compared to a normal saline treated group (23). Shoemaker et al. (24), have shown that plasma infusion is more effective than crystalloid for the improvement of cardiac output. Since capillary permeability to albumin is increased dramatically during the first 24 hours post burn, a significant amount of administered albumin will migrate into the interstitial space. Therefore the administration of albumin during the first 24 hours post burn should be restricted to a maximum of 12.5 g/liter in the infusion fluid.

In the first several days after injury and periodically thereafter if necessary, Larson and Wells (25) also suggest the use of albumin to maintain a serum albumin concentration higher than 20 g/liter. However, hyperalimentation is mandatory and should be instituted in the early stage. For the otherwise healthy patients with burns up to 30% of the body surface, there is no indication to use albumin. So in burns, albumin administration is inappropriate (standard 9) if:

1. less than 30% of the body surface is burned,
2. more than 30% of the body surface is burned, but the average albumin concentration in the infusion fluids is more than 12.5 g/liter during the first 24 hrs. post burn,
3. in the following 5 days if serum albumin is above 20 g/liter, or if serum albumin is below 20 g/liter and no hyperalimentation is instituted.

The pre- and postoperative care of patients in a catabolic state with protein-deficiency, should include primarily adequate alimentation (gastric-tube feeding, jejunostomy or intravenous hyperalimentation) with at least 2000 Calories and a sufficient amount of amino acids. Preoperative hyperalimentation, as shown by Holter and Fisher is very effective in significantly increasing serum albumin concentration and markedly decreasing postoperative weight loss (26). Albumin infusion should only be used when serum concentrations of albumin or protein are lower than 25 g/liter and 52 g/liter respectively (27) (colloid osmotic pressure = 20 mm torr) (standard 10). For patients with ARDS, this critical level of serum albumin or protein should be higher (35 g/liter and 60 g/liter respectively). In this regard, it is important to mention that attempts to raise serum protein concentration higher than 60 g/liter in notable catabolic patients, even with massive doses of albumin, have proved to be useless (27).

In the studies of Tullis (27) and Hoye et al. (23), it has been demonstrated that very extensive operations can result in a loss of 30 to 80% of the total circulating albumin mass. For such patients albumin infusion in the immediate post-operative period may be very useful. However if the main purpose of albumin administration is to improve an oncotic deficit, albumin should be given only in the first 48 hrs. after the operation, and in general only to patients with very extensive operations (for example pancreatico-duodenectomy) or in high-risk patients with extensive operations (standard 11). In patients undergoing a cardio-pulmonary bypass, the pump-priming solution is adequate when the albumin concentration is 25 g/liter and the hemoglobin concentration is 20 g/liter (27) (standard 12).

In summary there is an inappropriate use of albumin or plasma infusion if:

1. serum albumin concentration is $\geq$ 40 g/liter,

2. more than 4 units of albumin 20% (125 ml units) are given in 24 hrs., and no remarkable external loss of albumin is present,
3. the patient has inoperable cancer,
4. no clear indication is present (none of those stated below),
5. in ARDS one of the above standards 1, 2 or 3 is present,
6. in high-risk patients (older than 70 years, or with severe intercurrent disease or with pulmonary contusion or head trauma) in shock, one of the standards 1, 2 or 3 is also present,
7. in adult otherwise healthy patients with hemorrhagic shock resuscitation does not start with 3000 ml of crystalloid and 1000 ml of haemacel or dextran solution,
8. in adult otherwise healthy patients with septic shock in early stage, as mentioned in standard 7,
9. in burn shock:
   - less than 30% of the body surface is burned,
   - more than 30% of the body surface is burned, but the average albumin concentration of infusion fluids used during the first 24 hrs. is more than 12.5 g/liter,
   - in the following 5 days the serum albumin concentration is above 20 g/liter or if serum albumin is below 20 g/liter and no hyperalimentation is instituted,
10. for the undernutrition of a surgical patient, no (hyper-) alimentation is instituted with at least 2000 calories and a sufficient amount of amino acids or if adequate (hyper-) alimentation is instituted but the serum albumin is higher than 25 g/liter or serum protein is more than 52 g/liter,
11. the use of albumin is to provide for a postoperative oncotic deficit, if the operation is not very extensive or extensive in a high risk patient, or if albumin infusion is given longer than the first 48 hrs. after surgery,
12. in cardio-pulmonary bypass, the pump-priming solution contains albumin more than 25 g/liter.

To verify the use and abuse of albumin according to these standards, we have performed a retrospective study in all patients who had albumin or plasma protein infusions from 1-1-77 to 31-7-77 and were admitted to our department of general surgery. It should be emphasized that such standards did not exist during the period of stydy. If multiple abuses occurred in the same patient, only the most obvious abuse was notified. If none of the stated indications or standards was presen, the patient's case was referred to standard 4. This includes low blood pressure after operation, ileus or loss of ascitic fluid.

The utilization of albumin in the emergency room, during anaesthesia and in the intensive care unit is not included in this study. However, some data concerning albumin administration in the traumatology unit are available. During the study period, 7262 patients have been admitted and 62 had serious multiple injuries. Of those 62 patients, 6 required more than 4000 ml of infusion fluids before cross-matches blood was available and 3 others belonged to the high risk group. Thus a total of 9 patients probably needed albumin during their admission according to the established standards (15% of the multiple-injury patients). The total amount of albumin and plasma protein used in the department of traumatology during this period of study was 118 units (Table 1). It can, therefore, be concluded

Table 1. Units of colloid solution used for infusion during the period from 1-1-1977 to 31-7-1977

	Albumin (125 ml/unit)	Plasma protein (250 ml/unit)	Haemaccel (500 ml/unit)	Dextran-sol. (500 ml/unit)	Total
General surgery	446	121	–	–	567
Trauma	33	85	132	10	260

that there was probably no major abuse of albumin in the emergency room in trauma cases.

During the 7 month period of study, 552 patients have been admitted to a general surgical ward of 64 beds. 60 patients (10.8%) have had albumin or plasma protein infusion with a total use of 567 units during this period (± 9.5 units per patient). One patient is excluded from further analysis because this patient alone had received 129 units of albumin (22.8% of the total use). He is a 72 year old male with multiple small intestinal fistulas, complicating a surgically curative Bricker operation performed in an irradiated abdomen. He still remained in the ward during the complete period of study and had continuously intravenous hyperalimentation. In this period, three laparotomies have been performed to close or drain the fistulas. Based on the established standards he should be included in the "use" group (standard 10), but this would bias all further data. Therefore, 59 patients and 438 units of albumin are left for further analysis. As shown in Table 2, the most important abuse of albumin is found in association with

Table 2. Appropriate and inappropriate use of albumin and plasma protein infusions in a general surgical ward (1-1-1977 to 31-7-1977)

Standard	Appropriate use: Number of patients	Number of units	Average units per patient	Inappropriate use: Number of patients	Number of units	Average units per patient
1. Serum-albumin $\geq$ 40 g/l				3	24	8.0
2. > 4 units in 24 hrs.				1	17	
3. Inoperable cancer				6	115	19.2
4. No apparent reason				14	51	3.6
5. ARDS	3	13	4.3			
6. High risk[b] and shock	3	23	7.7			
7. Hem. shock[c]	0	0		2	4	
8. Septic shock[c]	0	0		1	1	
9. Burn shock[c]	0	0		0	0	
10. Undernutrition, operation, and adeq. alimentation[c]	8	60	7.5	0	0	
11. Postoperative oncotic deficit[c]	4	13	3.2	14	117	8.4
Subtotal	18	109	6.0	41	329	8.0
One patient (standard 10) excluded from study	1	129				
	19	238	12.5	41	329	8.0

[a] 1 Unit of albumin: 125 ml of 20% albumin solution.
 1 Unit of plasma protein: 250 ml of pasteurized plasma solution (protein content 3.8%; 95% albumin).
[b] High risk: 70 years or older, severe intercurrent disease, pulmonary contusion or head trauma.
[c] Standards for inappropriate use: see text.

standards 3 and 11. Patients with inoperable cancer have received a total of 115 units or 26.2% of the total use. The average number of units used per patient of this group was the highest ($\pm$ 19.2 units/per patient). The utilization of albumin in postoperative patients probably intended to substitute for an oncotic deficit, was also a frequent source of abuse: 117 units in total or 26.7% of the total use. A substantial number of patients in both groups would clearly have benefited from adequate alimentation. The mean serum protein concentration in these two groups was 59 g/liter (normal 60–80 g/liter). In comparing the "use" group to the "abuse group" it is interesting to note that the average use of albumin in the abuse group was higher ($\pm$ 8 units/patient) than in the use group ($\pm$ 6 units/patient) (Table 3).

From this study, it is apparent that all by all, 329 units (75.1% of total use) could have been spared without harm to the patient, if one adhered to a number of generally acceptable standards (Table 3).

Table 3. Total use and inappropriate use of albumin and plasma-protein infusions (1-1-1977 to 31-7-1977).

	Number of patients	Number of units	Average units/patient
Appropriate use	18 (30.5%)	109 (24.9%)	6.0
Inappropriate use	41 (69.5%)	329 (75.1%)	8.0
Total	59 patients	438	± 7.4

SUMMARY

A number of standards concerning the use and abuse of albumin in acute clinical conditions is suggested and discussed. These standards are established not on strictly theoretical background, but rather on clinical common sense. Therefore, they can probably be considered as general acceptable guidelines for albumin use in acute clinical conditions. To verify the use and abuse of albumin according to these standards, a retrospective study was performed in 59 patients who were admitted in our department and had albumin treatment.

Application of the standards for abuse of albumin could have resulted in an economy of 75.1% of the total albumin use.

REFERENCES

1. Kunin CM: Audits of antimicrobial usage. Veterans Administration ad hoc interdisciplinary advisory Committee on Antimicrobial Drug Usage. JAMA 237:1003–1008, 1977.
2. Fulton RL, Jones CE: The cause of posttraumatic pulmonary insufficiency in man. Surg Gynecol Obstet 140:179–186, 1975.
3. Browdie DA, Deane R, Shinozaki T, et al: Adult respiratory distress syndrome, sepsis and extra-corporeal membrane oxygenation. J Trauma 17:579–586, 1977.
4. Skillman JJ, Bushnell LS, Hedley-Whyte J: Peritonitis and respiratory failure after abdominal operations. Ann Surg 170:122–127, 1969.
5. Powers SR: Shock and metabolism. Surg Gynecol Obstet 140:211–215, 1975.
6. Lundsgaard-Hansen P: Oncotic deficit and albumin treatment. Proceedings of the Workshop on Albumin, February 12–13, 1975. Publication no 76–925. National Heart and Lung Institute, National Institutes of Health, Dept of Health, Education and Welfare, Bethesda, Md 242–252, 1975.
7. Moss GS: Fluid distribution after dilutional hemo-expansion. Surg Forum 19:19–21, 1968.
8. Goris RJA: Natriumlactaat en bloedverlies. Ned Tijdschr Geneesk 114:2113–2115, 1970.
9. Michalsky AH, Lowenstein E, Austen WG, et al: Patterns of oxygenation and cardio-

vascular adjustment to acute, transient normovolemic anemia. Ann Surg 168:946–956, 1968.
10. Cooper JD, Maeda M, Lowenstein E: Lung water accumulation with acute hemodilution in dogs. J Thorac Cardiovasc Surg 69:957–965, 1975.
11. Zarins CK, Rice CL, Smith DE, et al: Role of lymphatics in preventing hypooncotic pulmonary edema. Surg Forum 27:257–259, 1976.
12. Skillman JJ, Restall DS, Salzman EW: Randomized trial of albumin vs electrolyte solutions during abdominal aortic operations. Surgery 78:291–303, 1975.
13. Laks H, O'Connor NE, Anderson W, et al: Crystalloid versus colloid hemodilution in man. Surg Gynecol Obstet 142:506–512, 1976.
14. Siemens R, Polk HC, Gray LA, et al: Indications for thoracotomy following penetrating thoracic injury. J Trauma 17:493–500, 1977.
15. Lowe RJ, Moss GS, Jilek J, et al: Crystalloid vs colloid in the etiology of pulmonary failure after trauma: a randomized trial in man. Surgery 81: 676–683, 1977.
16. Cloutier CT, Lowery BD, Carey LC: The effect of hemodilutional resuscitation on serum-protein levels in humans in hemorrhagic shock. J Trauma 9: 514–521, 1969.
17. Virgilio RW, Smith DE, Rice CL, et al: Effect of colloid osmotic pressure and pulmonary capillary wedge pressure on intrapulmonary shunt. Surg Forum 27:168–170, 1976.
18. Gump FE, Kinney JM, Iles M, et al: Duration and significance of large fluid loads administered for circulatory support. J Trauma 10:431–439, 1970.
19. Holcroft JW, Trunkey DD, Carpenter MA: Sepsis in the Baboon: factors affecting resuscitation and pulmonary edema in animals resuscitated with Ringers lactate versus plasmanate. J Trauma 17:600–610, 1977.
20. Monafo WW: The treatment of burn shock by the intravenous and oral administration of hypertonic lactated saline solution. J Trauma 10:575–586, 1970.
21. Moylan JA, Reckler JM, Mason AD: Resuscitation with hypertonic lactated saline in thermal injury. Am J Surg 125:580–584, 1973.
22. Fox CL, Stanford JW: Comparitive efficacy of hypo-, iso- and hypertonic sodium solutions in experimental burn shock. Surgery 75:71–79, 1974.
23. Shimazaki S, Toshiharu Y, Tanaka N et al: Body fluid changes during hypertonic lactated saline solution therapy for burn shock. J Trauma 17:38–43, 1977.
24. Shoemaker WC, Matsuda T, State D: Relative hemo-dynamic effectiveness of whole blood and plasma expanders in burned patients. Surg Gynecol Obstet 144:909–914, 1977.
25. Larson DL, Wells CH: Plasma protein shifts in thermal injury. Proceedings of the Workshop on Albumin, February 12–13, 1975. Publication no 76–925. National Heart and Lung Institute, National Institutes of Health, Dept of Health, Education and Welfare, Bethesda, Md 221–227, 1975.
26. Holter AR, Fisher JE: The effects of perioperative hyperalimentation on complications in patients with carcinoma and weight loss. J Surg Res 23:31–34, 1977.
27. Tullis JL: Albumin.2. Guidelines for clinical use. JAMA 237:460–463, 1977.
28. Hoye RC, Bennett SH, Geelhoed GW, et al: Fluid volume and albumin kinetics occurring with major surgery. JAMA 222:1255–1261, 1972.

14. Use and abuse of albumin and plasma protein infusions in chronic protein depletion

C.B.H.W. Lamers

Chronic protein depletion is mostly reflected in hypoproteinemia. All protein fractions can be reduced but a decreased serum albumin level, which forms the bulk of serum protein, is most prominent. This depressed serum albumin concentration can be the result of 1) an impaired synthesis; 2) an increased loss or degradation; 3) an altered distribution or 4) a combination of factors (1). Albumin has proved to be not essential to human life since patients with analbuminemia are without important symptoms (2). The functions of albumin are firstly to maintain plasma colloid osmotic pressure and secondly to bind and to transport several substances like metals, ions, fatty acids, drugs, hormones, bilirubin, metabolites, etc. (3). Hypoalbuminemia is not a disease in itself, but like for example a raised E.S.R., fever or weight loss, merely a symptom of a disease. Symptoms of a disease should only be treated if they are dangerous or troublesome to the patient. Obviously, the underlying disorder has to be treated as vigorously as possible. A favorable effect of such a treatment will often be reflected in increasing serum albumin levels.

According to data from the Memorial Sloan-Kettering Cancer Center, 17% of the albumin supply was administered to patients with chronic protein deficiency as a result of protein-losing gastroenteropathy, nephrosis, hepatic cirrhosis or malabsorption, while 15% was given to patients with debilitating diseases (4). These data can probably be extrapolated to many other hospitals.

Because of the shortage and expense of albumin, the indications for albumin infusion in patients with hypoalbuminemia should be well-considered.

Hypoalbuminemia can result in a depressed colloid osmotic pressure of plasma, which in turn can lead to edema and a contracted intravascular volume, that subsequently stimulates the renin-angiotensin system and aldosteron secretion (5). Very potent diuretics have been developed in recent years which, when given in adequate doses in addition to salt restriction, will markedly reduce edema in almost every patient.

What are at present the indications for albumin infusion in chronic hypoalbuminemia? Let us consider the most frequent disorders accompanied by chronic hypoalbuminemia successively.

NEPHROTIC SYNDROME

Urinary protein loss in nephrotic patients can lead to severe hypoalbuminemia with massive edema and a contracted intravascular volume. It has been shown that infusion of albumin can result in an increase in plasma colloid osmotic pressure, a reduction of edema and to a rise in plasma volume, in glomerular filtration rate and in urinary excretion of water and sodium (6, 7). This favorable effect of the intravenous administration of albumin, however, is of very limited duration, since massive urinary loss of albumin adversely affects the net therapeutical result (6, 7). Salt restriction in combination with powerful diuretics should be preferred to albumin infusions in the symptomatic treatment of patients with nephrotic syndrome. In a few patients, however, diuretics are ineffective or the dose to be administered has to be limited because of side-effects, such as postural hypotension, azotemia or hyponatremia (8). It has recently been shown that albumin infusions administered in combination with diuretics can induce urinary excretion of sodium and water followed by resolution of edema in patients who were previously refractory to diuretics or had developed severe dose-limiting side-effects (8). Administration of albumin should be restricted to nephrotic patients, in whom diuretic treatment has proved to be insufficiently effective.

HEPATIC CIRRHOSIS

Patients with cirrhosis of the liver have often low serum albumin levels, which can lead to edema and can contribute to the formation of ascites. Peripheral edema in cirrhotic patients can generally be treated by salt restriction and diuretics, and albumin infusions although being effective are rarely needed. The symptomatic treatment of ascites, however, is much more difficult. The small difference between the colloid osmotic pressure of plasma and ascitic fluid and the high portal pressure are important factors in the formation and maintenance of ascites (9, 10). Infusion of albumin, unfortunately, raises not only the colloid osmotic pressure of plasma but also of the ascitic fluid in a parallel manner (9, 10). Moreover, infusion of albumin induced an increase in intrasplenic pressure, representing the splanchnic capillary pressure, in about half of the patients studied by Losowsky and Atkinson (9). This rise in intrasplenic pressure was most prominent in those patients who had a high pressure previous to albumin infusion (9). Furthermore, these studies showed that infusion of albumin could reduce ascitic volume in patients with a low plasma colloid osmotic pressure in whom ascites had developed with only moderate portal hypertension. In patients with ascites accompanied by a high intrasplenic pressure, however, infusion of albumin led to a further rise of this pressure and subsequently to an increase in ascitic volume (9). Since salt restriction and diuretics usually induce a reduction in plasma volume, ascitic fluid will move into the vascular space to restore effective plasma volume. Therefore, this treatment is often effective in reducing ascitic volume. Very high doses of diuretics being required in some patients with massive ascites may lead to adverse reactions, such as postural hypotension, hyponatremia, azotemia and increasing encephalopathy (11). These patients can be treated by abdominal paracentesis. As pointed out by Knauer and Lowe (12), removal of less than 1500 ml of ascitic fluid will not result in a decrease of cardiac output. However, removal of many liters of ascites in cirrhotic patients is contraindicated, because it results in pronounced protein loss and a severe fall in circulating volume, precipitating encephalopathy (11). Ultrafiltration of ascitic fluid and reinfusion of the protein richer and salt-poorer ascitic concentrate is the treatment of choice in patients who have proved to be resistent to diuretics or have shown considerable side-effects (11). This therapy results in a reduction of ascites and in an increase in urinary excretion of sodium and water. This procedure should be combined with or followed by diuretic treatment to prevent rapid reaccumulation of ascitic fluid (13, 14). Recently, a subcutaneous peritoneovenous shunt has also proved to be effective in the symptomatic treatment of ascites (15). Furthermore, it has been shown that prolonged therapy with albumin has no favorable effect on the general condition, the diuretic needs or the ultimate prognosis of patients with hepatic cirrhosis (16). It has been suggested that administration of albumin may precipitate bleeding from esophageal varices by increasing portal pressure (16, 17).

PROTEIN-LOSING GASTRO-ENTEROPATHY

Increased protein loss from the gastrointestinal tract can result in hypoal-buminemia (1, 18). The serum albumin level may be such low that edema occurs. This can mostly be adequately treated by salt restriction and diuretics. Infusion of albumin is therefore not indicated in the symptomatic treatment of such patients. Moreover, after infusion albumin will rapidly leak into the gastrointestinal tract.

MALNUTRITION

When malnutrition results in hypoalbuminemia, oral administration of protein or infusion of amino acids will induce an increase in serum albumin concentration. Tryptophan and the branched-chain amino acids seem to play an important role in stimulating the synthesis of albumin by the liver (19). Administration of albumin is an expensive and unjustified manner of supplying nutritional requirements. The breakdown of albumin is rather slow, having an half-life of about 20 days, and its contents of the essential amino acids methionine, isoleucine and notably tryptophan is poor (20).

OTHER CONDITIONS

Patients with chronic infections or malignancy often show low serum albumin levels. The mechanism of the hypoalbuminemia in these patients seems to be complex (1). When hypoalbuminemic edema occurs, treatment is not essentially different from that in patients with edema of other origin. It should be emphasized that an adequate intake of nutrients is very important in these patients being in a chronic catabolic state.

When rapid resolution of edema is urgently needed, the simultaneous use of salt restriction, diuretics and albumin infusion may be indicated. Davison et al. (8) found that this combination was highly effective in the treatment of gross edema in a nephrotic patient, who had recently under-gone appendectomy. Short term studies of Vlahcevic et al. (13) and

Eknoyan et al. (21) have also shown that the simultaneous therapy with diuretics and infusion of albumin or ascitic fluid in cirrhotic patients is superior to one of these treatments alone.

CONCLUSIONS

Infusions of albumin are of very restricted value in the symptomatic treatment of chronic protein depletion. The following indications are proposed.

- severe edema with resistance to salt restriction and diuretics,
- severe edema with important side-effects attributable to diuretics,
- urgent need for rapid resolution of edema,
- cirrhotic patients with ascites and extreme hypoalbuminemia.

It is emphasized that the administration of albumin should be combined with salt restriction and when possible with diuretics.

The use of protein infusions should be limited to correct transient and specific problems caused by hypoalbuminemia, which has proved to be resistant to other forms of treatment.

REFERENCES

1. Rothschild MA, Oratz M, Schreiber SS: Albumin metabolism. Gastroenterology 64:324–337, 1973.
2. Waldmann TA, Gordon RS, Rosse W: Studies on the metabolism of the serum proteins and lipids in a patient with analbuminemia. Am J Med 37:960–968, 1964.
3. Rosenoer VM: Clinical aspects of albumin metabolism. Albumin, structure, function and uses, Rosenoer VM, Oratz M, Rothschild MA (eds), Oxford-New York, Pergamon Press, 1977, pp 345–367.
4. Mayer K, Whitsett C: Albumin and plasma protein infusion in chronic protein deficiency or loss. Proceedings of the workshop on albumin, Feb. 12–13, 1975. Sgouris JT, René A, (eds), Publication no 76-925, National Institute of Health, Bethesda Md, pp 228–238.
5. Davison AM: The use of albumin concentrates in hypoproteinaemic states. Clinics in Haematology 5:135–148, 1976.
6. Luetscher JA, Hall AD, Kremer VL: Treatment of nephrosis with concentrated human serum albumin. I. Effects on the proteins of body fluids. J Clin Invest 28:700–712, 1949.
7. Luetscher JA, Hall AD, Kremer VL: Treatment of nephrosis with concentrated human serum albumin. II. Effects on renal function and on excretion of water and some electrolytes. J Clin Invest 29:896–904, 1950.
8. Davison AM, Lambie AT, Verth AH, et al: Salt-poor albumin in management of nephrotic syndrome. Br Med J 1:481–484, 1974.
9. Losowsky MS, Atkinson M: Intravenous albumin in the treatment of diuretic-resistant ascites in portal cirrhosis. Lancet 2: 386–389, 1961.

10. Mankin H, Lowell A: Osmotic factors influencing the formation of ascites in patients with cirrhosis of the liver. J Clin Invest 27:145–153, 1948.
11. Parbhoo SP, Ajdukiewicz A, Sherlock S: Treatment of ascites by continuous ultra-filtration and reinfusion of protein concentrate. Lancet 1:949–952, 1974.
12. Knauer CM, Lowe HM: Hemodynamics in the cirrhotic patient during paracentesis. N Engl J Med 276:491–496, 1967.
13. Vlahcevic ZR, Adham NF, Chalmers TC, et al: Intravenous therapy of massive ascites in patients with cirrhosis. I. Short-term comparison with diuretic treatment. Gastro-enterology 53:211–219, 1967.
14. Shear L, Ching, S, Gabuzda GJ: Compartmentalization of ascites and edema in patients with hepatic cirrhosis. N Engl J Med 282:1391–1396, 1970.
15. LeVeen HH, Wapnick S, Grosberg S, et al: Further experience with peritoneo-venous shunt for ascites. Ann Surg 184:574–581, 1976.
16. Wilkinson P, Sherlock S: The effect of repeated albumin infusions in patients with cirrhosis. Lancet 2:1125–1129, 1962.
17. Faloon WW, Eckhardt RD, Murphy TL, et al: An evaluation of human serum albumin in the treatment of cirrhosis of the liver. J Clin Invest 28:583–594, 1949.
18. Van Tongeren JHM et al: Causes of hypoalbuminemia. This volume, p 117.
19. Yap SH, Hafkenscheid JCM, van Tongeren JHM, et al: Rate of synthesis of albumin in relation to serum levels of essential amino acids in patients with bacterial over-growth in the small bowel. Eur J Clin Invest 4:279–284, 1974.
20. Tullis JL: Albumin 2. Guidelines for clinical use. JAMA 237:460–463, 1977.
21. Eknoyan G, Martinez-Maldonado M, Yium JJ, et al: Combined ascitic-fluid and furosemide infusion in the management of ascites. N Engl J Med 282:713–717, 1970.

Index